MW00975522

Life is Healing School of Qigong
The 5 Yin Organs Taoist Medical Qigong
with Optional DVD Level 1

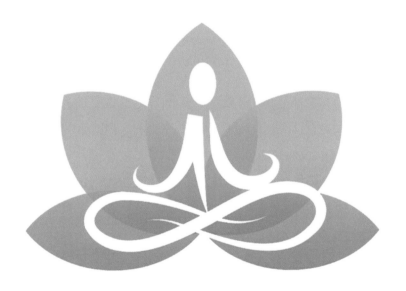

Following the detail instructions in this guide
will allow you to be able to practice Medical
Qigong correctly and understand how and when
it should be applied. We highly recommend that
you view our instructional DVD to help
facilitate your understanding and practice.

Medical Disclaimer
The information provided in this book is designed to provide helpful information on the subjects discussed. This book is not meant to be used, nor should it be used, to diagnose or treat any medical condition. For diagnosis or treatment of any medical problem, consult your own physician. The publisher and author are not responsible for any specific health or allergy needs that may require medical supervision and are not liable for any damages or negative consequences from any treatment, action, application or preparation, to any person reading or following the information in this book. References are provided for informational purposes only.

Brief Biography of Dr. Angelo Isom, ND, CHS, MQT

Dr. Angelo Isom, also known as Laoshur Muntu Isom is a graduate of New York University, Columbia University, Georgia State University and Clayton College of Natural Healing. He holds several degrees in various fields including psychology, philosophy, teaching methods, education and naturopathy and numerous other certifications. He is a male health advisor, researcher and coach.

Dr. Isom's experiences in healing encompass multiple areas of research and study. Some of these areas include acupuncture, qigong, yoga, internal martial arts, qigong and martial arts lineage holder, grounding, energy healing, human sexuality, western and eastern herbs, diet and nutrition, Chinese massage and health supplements.

Dr. Isom has been fortunate to study cultural healing methods and herbs while visiting such countries as Brazil, Mexico's Yucatan Peninsula, Haiti, Jamaica, Honduras, Saint Thomas Virgin Islands, Aruba, Curacao and Puerto Rico. Dr. Isom is CEO and Director of Life is Healing, a holistic wellness Institute. Over the years, he has counseled countless numbers of clients seeking to restore their health and achieve optimal fitness and health. Dr. Isom is the author of several books "The Sexual Warrior Within" copy written 2015 and "Are You Healthy Enough for Sex?" also, copy written 2015. Both books are available on amazon.com

Dr. Isom's approach to healing and rejuvenation focuses upon the cultivation of the 3 treasures known as Jing, Qi and Shen. He makes good use of The 5 Elements Theory combined with methods of grounding, internal cleansing, eating according to the seasons, mind/body balance to maintain and restore health. Dr. Isom enjoys biking, swimming, scuba diving, jazz guitar, science documentaries, traveling and conversing in Portuguese and Spanish. Dr. Angelo Isom, ND also known as Laoshur Muntu Isom is the chief master level instructor (Laoshur) for the Harmonizing Fist School of Martial Arts. He is also a professional member of the Chinese National Qigong Association and American Tai Chi and Qigong Association. These associations serve to create higher standards of practice for internal martial arts and qigong, the research of new methods and promoting of special events to share Qigong Healing worldwide.

Cathy Blackburn Brief Biography

Cathy is an avid practitioner of Bagua Zhang (similar to tai chi but more active) and a Certified Qigong Therapist/CQT. She is the co-founder of the Life is Healing Institute. Cathy has studied holistic health extensively under the tutelage of Dr. Angelo Isom N.D. (also known as Laoshur Muntu Isom) and is the author of her first book Cook, Eat and Lose which is available on amazon.

Through experimentation and years of research she has tested and perfected numerous food recipes that resulted in her loss of over 30 pounds in less than four months. The strategies that helped her to achieve this success was well documented in her recently published book. This extensive experience and broad spectrum of knowledge on healing modalities include: healthy lifestyle options with an emphasis on nutrition, exercise techniques that can fit into most lifestyles, herbal supplementation and essential oils.

Cathy is also a certified Aroma/Touch Therapist and Wellness Advocate with Do Terra International specializing in the therapeutic usage of essential oils. We provide ongoing classes that provide detailed information about how to incorporate the power of these oils into your lifestyle. These include their topical application, how to use them aromatically, internally and for household cleaning.

Cathy practices meditation, she loves communing with nature, bike riding, vigorous walks, high intensity training (HIT), Qigong, traveling and preparing healthy meals, speaks Spanish and Portuguese. Cathy is an advocate for healthier lifestyle choices and enjoys sharing this powerful information with others that are on the same path and want to change their life.

Why Qigong is Important to Me?

I am very passionate about Qigong and internal martial arts. These arts have played an important part in my health and well-being. I am committed to these arts and have experienced the benefits of consistent practice firsthand. Qigong has given me more flexibility, deeper breathing and the ability to feel the qi throughout my body. Every time I practice, I feel totally alive. My deepest wish is for you to experience this for yourself. I realized as I grew older that I had several choices to make.

One: I could be proactive by choosing a healthier lifestyle, make better dietary choices and exercise more. I realized that I was the only one who could make these goals a reality.

Two: I could depend on others to make critical decisions for me that may or may not be in my best interest.

Three: I could choose to simply ignore my physical, emotional and spiritual needs and take the easy way out by not doing anything.

My enlightened choice was to be proactive by taking charge of my health. This was a win- win situation for me as well as my loved ones.

I highly recommend that you make Qigong part of your lifestyle so that you too can reap the benefits of optimal radiant health.

Favorite Quotes:

"Self-care is not selfish. You cannot serve from an empty vessel."
-Eleanor Brown

"Motivation may be what starts you off, but it's habit that keeps you going back for more. Are your habits working for you or against you? Are your habits helping you to achieve your goals or hindering the process?"

---Miya Yamanouchi, Embrace Your Sexual Self: A Practical Guide for Women

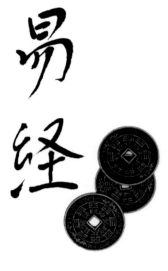

Good Luck and Prosperity Coin

Author's Personal Note:

It is only truthful to say that I consider myself to be both a student and teacher of Qigong after being privileged to practice this art for over 35 years. Special thanks go to some of my most notable teachers
 Sifu Raymond Nelson – who introduced me to Qigong, Tiger Claw and Mantis martial arts, Kurt Baker, Steve Cottrell and Jason Lau whom all helped me to refine my Wing Chun Concepts. Special recognition to Grandmaster Chiu Leun - 7 Star Mantis, his disciple Raymond Ming Loy – Mantis, Master
Khallid Hakim- who taught me deeper aspects of Taoist Qigong, Tai Ji, Bagua and Xing-Yi, Dr. Kam Yuen- who introduced me to Chinese Energetic Medicine and Shou-Yu Liang –who instructed me on the fine points of Tai Ji and Taoist Qigong.

My intimate and intuitive understanding of Qigong was the result of many years of training with martial arts masters, careful observations, and personal practice, testing trials, personal healings and inner energetic alchemy.
I also give much credit and thanks to all those ascended masters who have guided me during my meditative practice with spiritual insights and mental downloads of true knowledge and wisdom.

 During the course of my training I became aware that the only true reality that exists is the reality of the self and our degree of conscious awakening. The practice of Qigong is as much of spiritual journey as it is physical. Both the outer world of form and our physical 3D bodies operate primarily on the principles of duality or yin and yang. The original oneness and truth is called The Tao in China or Maat in Africa where there exists no duality but only divine perfection and harmony between heaven and earth and communal love.

As we think and visualize ourselves our reality begins to change. We truly live in a holographic world made up of thought and energy. Nothing is really solid. Reality in itself is not fixed but is malleable to conscious will and thought and sometimes to the thought of others. In order to practice Qigong correctly we must learn how to creatively visualize our physical and holographic bodies as a collective energy matrix projected by our will. We are all conductors of universal energy whether we know it or not. This energy adapts and modulates itself in accordance with our inner visualization and projection of intent.

How we visualize our holographic body as being healthy or ill directly or sometimes indirectly impacts our health based upon the law of attraction. Our holographic bodies are the blueprint for our physical makeup. Therefore, as we think so shall we manifest. You are only as healthy as you portray yourself in your mind. Changing this mental image of ourselves can ultimately change how we manifest our health. Our bodies respond to our mental subconscious thought even more than conscious thought. One of the key principles of Qigong healing states that where the mind goes qi flows.

My Favorite Quotes:
"Does life change you or do you change your life?"
(Dr. Wu Dhi)

"We know what we are but not what we may be."
 (Author unknown)

"Decide if you want to be well known or know something well."
(Dr. Angelo Isom)

What is the sound of one hand clapping?
(Zen Koan)
Answer: There is none!
Reflection: The sound of 1 hand clapping is merely a thought that must be made silent. In silence, we hear what cannot be heard. In silence, we hear our true self. In thought we hear chatter and are confused by what is and what is not. Therefore, 1 hand should never stop clapping and we should never stop listening to ourselves.
(My own personal wisdom and realization)
Reflection for You the Reader
How can you make a mirror by polishing a brick?"
(Zen Koan)

Why I Prefer Qigong Over Regular Exercises?

The reason why I devote much of my time to practicing Qigong exercises rather than the norm, like sports, running, tennis, weight lifting is not only to keep my body strong and flexible but to keep the flow of qi running through my energetic pathways or meridians. Longevity is a long- term health project. The reality is the comparison of long term health gains versus short term athletic success.

I recommend that if you choose to practice western external exercises then do so in a non-competitive manner with moderation. Qigong can still benefit an athlete by helping them reduce their recovery period, increase flexibility, better mental control and breathing endurance. After about one month of Qigong training, athletes learn how to relax more before a stressful event while using creative visualization and better posture to achieve their goals.

If you are not training to be an athlete, then keep it simple. Be mindful that western athletic training usually requires tremendous energy expenditure to achieve physical results such as bulking muscles and body sculpting or breaking records. Accumulating large muscles and body sculpting does not signify you are healthy. The process of reaching these fitness goals requires long hours of intense training, weird diets, high maintenance, long recovery and inflammation. The real downside can be seen from a long-term perspective of conditioning versus deconditioning.

Deconditioning occurs when an exercise is suspended for a period of 10 days or 2 weeks. During this period, an athlete can quickly lose many of the benefits he or she worked hard for over the course of months and years. These short- term gains that only leads to a long-term losses if the rigor of training is interrupted. In comparison, Qigong gives us long term gain with minimum short term setbacks. There are forms of Qigong most suitable for almost everyone. For example, if you are interested in building physical strength and toughening the body then the practice of Muscle Tendon Change and or Iron Shirt Qigong is right for you. Other Internal exercises and martial arts such as Tai Ji Chuan, Bagua Zhang and Xing-I can greatly assist in keeping the flow of energy balanced through the meridians. What does this mean for you? The answer is, a longer and healthier fit life, more awareness, a better functioning brain, optimal hormonal profile, stronger sexual appetite and peace of mind. If you are reading this manual, then you too have already join me in my quest to help spread this wisdom along with many other enlightened students that already are experiencing the benefits of:

The 5 Yin Organs Taoist Medical Qigong.

Qigong, pronounced as Chee Gung or Chi Kong, is a traditional powerful Chinese energy medicine art and science combining breathing, gentle movement, and meditation to cleanse, strengthen, and circulate energy (Qi). It was once known as Dao Yin, The Cultivating of Qi. It will bring you better health, vitality, and a longer, happier life.

"Qi" means vital energy of the body, and "Gong" means the skill and achievement cultivated through regular and disciplined practice. This is equal to Energy Work. Qigong is part of Traditional Chinese Medicine (TCM), which works with the Qi as a key feature of human psychology, physiology, and biology for healing and improving one's health and longevity. Qigong has been practiced with proven results in China for thousands of years and has many different forms.

According to some statistics, there are over 100,000 styles of Qigong in China today from Buddhism, Taoism, Confucian, and Kung Fu. The different styles have been created for different purposes. Qigong can be used in almost every aspect of life, making it a lot more rewarding with lesser symptoms of body, mind and spirit. In China, Qigong practices are revered as one of the ancient secrets to longevity and were traditionally only taught to royalty and their families. Meditation is also an important part of Qigong practice known as Shen gong, or spiritual work. Later, Qigong training was brought to Japan and became Zen meditation.

Some believe the Japanese version of Qigong is most likely Reiki. Meditation is a necessary training to direct the mind and regulate the Qi flow in the body. Once the energy is cultivated, it must be coordinated with the activities of the mind, body and spirit, so that mind and body can benefit from the synchronization and mutual influence. Training in meditation enables one to perceive the subtle levels at which the Qi functions, both at the level of the mind, body and spirit.

Dr. Isom's Personal Healing Story

As I recall, it was the year 2003 late August just before Labor Day. I had just moved into my new house and was quite excited about unpacking and decorating my home. There were quite a number social activities going on in Atlanta that weekend so I decided to go out and celebrate with some friends. We visited several clubs and ate dinner out. At about 5 am in the morning I was totally exhausted and decided to call it quits, go home and sleep. I slept to about 11:30 am the next day and upon waking I noticed that I had a strange sensation of numbness throughout my body. When I tried to get out of bed my body was unable to activate my muscles to move. I felt paralyzed with a numbness and tingling sensation all over my body. I struggled with my arms and eventually was able to get out of bed on to my feet.

I immediately noticed that I could barely feel my feet. It was at this point that I knew something was wrong. A friend called my doctor who recommended that I be rushed to the hospital by ambulance. After arriving at the hospital, the emergency doctors quickly sent me to the MRI for evaluation. My MRI revealed that I had a noticeable size lesion on my spinal cord in the cervical neck area. I was then diagnosed with a rare case of Transverse-Myletis Spinal Lesion. My neurologists were baffled as how I contracted this condition overnight.

Their best guess was based on a viral agent. In my case the actual cause was unknown. I was then prescribed and given anti-inflammatory, and antiviral medication. Both medications were ineffective in relieving my condition. My prognosis at this point seemed bleak. Both of my neurologists stated that I would be permanently disabled and needed to make preparation for the worst. They also said that there was no known cure and that spinal nerves don't grow back once damaged. I asked myself, how could this happen to me, especially since I was only 51 years old. Shortly after that, I became angry, depressed and confused.

I thought about my conditions for several days and decided that I could heal myself. Prior to this incident, I did practice martial arts for self-defense but didn't focus on Qi Gong for healing and balance. I then made a commitment to myself to heal using my previous knowledge and belief of Qigong as a healing art.

I started with deep breathing and gradually progressed to standing arm swaying movements. Over the course of the next two days I noticed a slight improvement in the sensation in my legs and feet. It was at this point I began to walk slowly with better balance.

I upgraded my Qigong practice to the Bagua Circle Walking method I had learned several years prior. For those who don't know, Bagua is a Chinese internal martial art that emphasizes the use of circle walking, spiral energetic movements done with meditative focus. I religiously practiced this method for 1 hour every day for 6 days a week. After about a week I could feel my legs and feet becoming stronger with more nerve sensations. I persisted another week and then notice that I could move more freely. The third week was my breakthrough week. Most the numbing sensations had gradually subsided. It was at this point that I felt so encouraged and optimistic about having a full recovery.

After about a month I made an appointment for another MRI. This time the results were unbelievable to my neurologist. He told me that my spinal nerves had regenerated and had weaved themselves back to normal. He stated that the good news was that I no longer had a lesion on my spine and my recovery was miraculous. My neurologist told me that whatever I was doing to keep at it.

After about three months I returned to work and was pleased to know that I no longer was eligible for permanent disability payments.
Wow, that was great news for me since most people do not ever recover from Transverse-Myletis Spinal Lesions. My only secret was the daily practice of Qigong and a positive attitude towards healing. Qigong gave me life to change my life. Truly a blessing unfolded.

Table of Contents

Chapter 1

The Cycles of Life

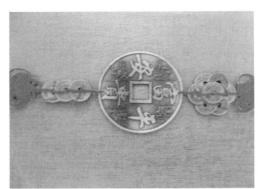

Good Fortune and Longevity Coin

The cycle of life flows from Wu Chi or the void > to Tai Ji or Yin and Yang > to 5 Elements Energy and continues to the Bagua or 8 Changes of life. Within these cycles are a myriad of permutations and transformations. The life cycle for a man is renewed every 7 years and based upon the solar cycle. Unlike men, women have a 8 year life period heavily influenced by the lunar cycle.

Yin and Yang Cycles can affect us hourly, daily, weekly, monthly and yearly. Our bodies experiences seasonal cycles and require us to make energetic adjustments via diet, activity, thought and mindset. Qigong can help us stay tuned in to these cycles while making needed adjustments in our life force to remain healthy.

There are two primary cycles that govern the flow of life. They are referred to as the Controlling or Destructive Cycle and the Creative Cycle. The Creative Cycle refers to the ability of one element being used to help create another. A good example of this is that wood is needed to make fire, fire is used to create earth or ash while earth creates minerals and metals. The flow of this energy eventually leads back to the creation of wood itself. The Controlling Cycle describes how one element is used to suppress another. For example, Fire can be controlled by water, water can control earth and metal is controlled by fire. These are just a few examples of these cycles. From a Qigong perspective, these elements also represent various types of energy in our body and the energy of seasonal change.

The 5 Element Cosmology Chart is based upon the Tai Ji Symbol

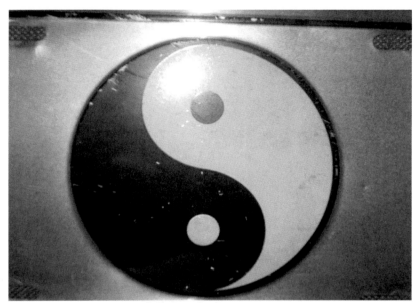
Tai Ji Symbol

The Taoist Masters of old realized that in order to be strong and healthy, humans need to have a balanced flow of qi and strong physical structure. Our organs, bones, cells and tissues need to be clean of toxins and full of free-flowing qi (life force) We also need to be able to stand on the ground in alignment with the forces of heaven and earth.

There are many forms of Qigong practices in existence today. The 3 major forms of Qigong are Medical/Healing, Martial Arts and Shen Gong or Spiritual Qigong. Some of these methods are quite practical and down to earth where as others are very esoteric, mysterious and impractical by modern standards. Most people today just don't have the time or luxury to do Qigong while trying to balance work, play, family and other responsibilities. This is one of the reasons I decided to create this manual guide.

Life Is Healing Qigong Instructional Manual will only focus only on the most practical and beneficial forms of Medical Qigong that almost anyone of

average or below average health, young or old can do. Medical Qigong was designed to balance and increase one's life force and healing potential. This form of Qigong should be part of everyone's health maintenance schedule of health. One of my own personal quote regarding consistency of practice states, "If it doesn't fit you will probably quit."
Therefore, it must be simple and beneficial to learn.

 Life is Healing Qigong is:
It is **easy** to learn and practice
It is **safe** to practice with no side-effects
It is **efficient** as it allows you to gather a large amount of Qi (energy) quickly and easily
It is **effective** and brings rapid positive results

 In addition to Qigong if you are interested in improving both your health and sex life without resorting to the use of steroids or medicines like Viagra or Cialis then and please refer to my following books, "The Sexual Warrior Within" and "Are You Healthy for Sex? By Dr. Angelo Isom. Both books are available on amazon. These books contain detail natural holistic strategies such as Qigong, tonic herbs, testosterone diet and life styles changes to optimize your health.

 The Life Is Healing Qigong Instructional Manual can be used as a reference manual guide to quickly find the best qigong posture/exercise to target your physical, mental or emotional health need. All the postures need not be done daily to improve health or build or cultivate qi.
Life Is Healing Qigong allows you to customize your routines, making it ideal for both the experienced practitioners and those new to qigong. One only needs to select 1 or more postures that are appropriate to your need at a particular time. All 5 of the postures can be practice daily if time permits.

 Qigong can be done seated, standing and in some cases lying down. The name of this method that will be presented in this manual is call,
The 5 Yin Organs Taoist Qigong Method based upon the ancient Taoist Chinese 5 Element Theory of health and wellness. This method stresses the tonification of the energy organ system in our body. It is my intent to present other forms of Qigong in future volume series to help further evolve your understanding of its potential benefits.

Where did Qigong Originate?

As far as it is known, Qigong first originated in Africa in the land of Kemet or ancient Egypt. Imhotep, known as the father of Egyptian medicine who preceded Hippocrates, understood the relationship of exercise, breathing and health. When the Chinese were just beginning to understand its importance, Imhotep clearly recognized that the unification of mind and body was a powerful form of medicine for healing in addition to herbs and minor surgery.

More on Imhotep:

Imhotep's best known writings were in his medical text. As a physician, Imhotep is believed to have been the author of the Edwin Smith Papyrus in which more than 90 anatomical terms and 48 injuries are described. He may have also founded a school of medicine in Memphis, a part of his cult center possibly known as "Asklepion, which remained famous for two thousand years. All of this occurred some 2,200 years before the western father of medicine Hippocrates was born.

Sir William Osler tells us that Imhotep was the first figure of a physician to stand out clearly from the mists of antiquity. Imhotep diagnosed and treated over 200 diseases, 15 diseases of the abdomen, 11 of the bladder, 10 of the rectum, 29 of the eyes, and 18 of the skin, hair, nails and tongue. Imhotep treated tuberculosis, gallstones, appendicitis, gout and arthritis. He also performed surgery and practiced some dentistry. Imhotep extracted medicine from plants. He also knew the position and function of the vital organs and circulation of the blood system. The Encyclopedia Britannica says, "The evidence afforded by Egyptian and Greek texts support the view that Imhotep's reputation was very respected in early times. His prestige increased with the lapse of centuries and his temples in Greek times were the centers of medical teachings."

This medical knowledge eventually was transplanted from Egypt to the Indus Valley which is now India and later organized into a system of health called Ayurvedic Medicine and Yoga. The word yoga literally means, the union of mind and body.

A reclusive priest known as Damo or Bodhidharma traveled from India across the Himalayan Mountains to China and introduced this new concept of healing and rejuvenation to the Shaolin Monastery. The Shaolin Monks practiced Qigong and gradually transformed it into Kung-Fu or martial arts. Many monks overtime migrated to a scared place call Wudan Mountain which later became the birthplace of the internal martial arts of Tai Ji Chuan, Hsing –I and Bagua Zhang. Martial arts started out as Qigong before it evolved to be what is now known as Kung-Fu.

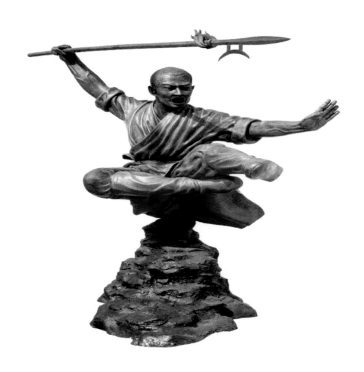

Chapter 2

What is Medical Qigong?

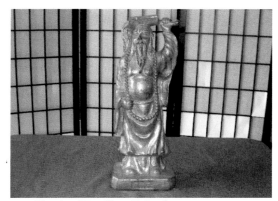
Taoist Healing Monk

Medical Qigong?

Qigong (pronounced chee-gung) is an ancient Chinese practice consisting of breathing exercises, flowing movement, creative visualization combined with meditation. It is truly the art of nourishing life. Done properly, it can revitalize the body and transform the spirit. Qigong helps to cultivate life force or qi for enhanced energy, radiant health and longevity. These benefits were known for thousands of years to the Chinese who help to preserve this healing art. Qigong is a spiritual and physical biofeedback system used to enhance radiant health. It literally means energy breath and cultivation skill. It is an ancient form of exercises and healing methods designed to heal specific body illnesses, channel life force energy, decrease aging, and raised the vibration of the body. Qigong is more than just a form of energy medicine. Many consider it to be form of an energy elixir that can nourish, replenish and strengthen the mind and body to increase longevity.

Qigong teaches us how to self-regulate, manipulate, circulate the daily flow of qi /life force into and out of our body to restore and maintain balanced emotional and physical well-being and vitality.
The practice of Qigong can assist us in dissolving blocked energy patterns that can lead to various organ dysfunctions, emotional crisis, symptoms of pain and weakness. It is one of the most natural forms of healing exercises to help almost anyone recover from accidental injuries or sport related injuries

due to athletic training or competition. Weightlifters, weekend warriors, runners, football players etc. all can benefit from Qigong training. The main goal of Qigong is to revitalize and replenish spent energy.

Medical Qigong is a branch of Traditional Chinese Medicine emerging as a cornerstone of many Eastern-influenced alternative medicine practices. Medical Qigong goes beyond self-cultivation, enlisting the assistance of a highly-trained and disciplined practitioner. Medical Qigong practitioners study and train for years, not only learning about the human anatomy and physiology, but cultivating their own energy through Qigong practice.

Medical Qigong can be used to address many common ailments or health concerns, including mental, physical or emotional stressors, physical pain, high blood pressure, headaches, anxiety or depression. Although ancient in origin, Qigong is a new category of exercise called Meditative Movement. From a physiological standpoint, Qigong practice puts the body into a state of relaxation and regeneration. This state is achieved by eliciting the Relaxation Response.

Medical Qigong also tends to focus more on the elongation of the spine using gentle rhythmic motions and massaging the internal organs. The deep abdominal breathing helps to massage the internal organs while increasing circulation of blood and spinal fluid. In order to be successful and healthy you must be first happy. One should strive to react with peace and joy to life's challenges in place of anger and fear. Stress and traumatic emotions can cause illnesses and rob the body of the vital life force known as Qi.

Illness is a physical, mental or emotional manifestation of an imbalance to be corrected. Medical Qigong Therapy relaxes the body, promotes the flow of qi, blood, oxygen, and nutrients to the cells of the body as well as the removal of waste products from the cells. The increase of qi flow by way of the microcirculation nourishes diseased or stressed tissues. The degree and speed of healing is heightened leading to a much shorter recovery time without side effects.

Recognizing excess or deficiency of energy in order to rebalance the body energetic system is one of the key the functional goals of Medical Qigong Therapy. Qigong is a way of life that focuses on creating and a balance of yin and yang known as Tai Ji while stimulating the development higher consciousness.

Life is Healing Qigong

- Prevent illness
- Assist in the recovery from illness if you have become unwell.
- Maintain a good level of day to day wellness
- Create outstanding health with regular, disciplined practice
- Elevate consciousness and build wisdom
- Build a happy, healthy and fulfilling life

Most active forms of Qigong utilize specific postures moving and still, breathing methods, guided imagery, sound and meditation principles to transform our mundane physical body into the body electric. The foundation of Kung-Fu is Qi Gong. It can increase the capacity for joy and peace by maintaining balance between the body, mind and emotions.
Medical Qigong also makes good use of specific postures, breathing, sound and visualizations to purge, tonify and balance the body. This is one of the safest and effective ways to rid the body matrix of toxic pathogens, emotional pain, and energy blocks that can cause mental and physical illness. Overtime one develops higher volume of what is known as the 3 treasures or San Bao. The three treasures are), Jing (hormones and vital fluids), Qi (energy) and Shen (spirit or higher consciousness). Qi is the medium between Jing/matter and Shen/Spirit that communicates how the life force energy interacts with our body.

Your Brain on Qigong

Qigong practice is good for your overall brain health and function. Regular practice of Qigong can entrain the brain to induce more alpha brain wave patterns or what is known as the super relax alert creative mindset. Alpha brain wave training is great for problem solving, new ideas, reflecting outside the box and a must for any artist.

Qigong practice allows the mind to enter deep into the body and target areas needing healing. Bilateral synchronization of the left and right brain hemisphere is made easier via the movements and breath coordination of Qigong. Enhanced production of vital brain neurotransmitters such as dopamine and serotonin are optimized for better brain health and mood with daily practice. The neuro- transmitter, Norepinephrine is also improved which can increase in the amount of oxygen going to our brain. which helps us think clearer and faster. Your brain is literally in the heaven zone when it's on Qigong. Consider it to be virtually a "Natural High Cocktail"

What is Qi and its Sources?

The term qi or chi is an umbrella translation that is cross cultural in scope. For example, in India it is called Prana, Ki or Reiki in Japan, Light/Spirit by Christians and Mana by Polynesians, Life Force or Bio-Energy by contemporary standards. The problem is that no one really understand understands exactly what qi but only what it appears to do or manifests. Without qi there is no life and where there is qi life exists. Within the concept of Qi there exist many form of it. An example of this is Wei Qi that protects the body from external invasion of cold, heat, dampness and Gu Qi that is derived from food and drinks.

 Nonliving objects can also store qi as well. Qi is literally everywhere. It can be derived from air, water, food, herbs, sound, light, grounding, trees, lakes, waterfall, mountains, holy places, animals and people etc. One just needs to know how to harness these energy sources.

Qi

"The vital essence of all things
It is this that brings them to life.
It generates the five grains below
And becomes the constellated stars above.
When flowing amid the heavens and the earth
We call it ghostly and numinous.
When installed within the chests of human beings,
We call them sages.
Therefore, this vital energy is:
Bright! - as if ascending the heavens;
Dark! - as if entering an abyss;
Vast! - as if dwelling in an ocean;
Lofty! - as if dwelling on a mountain peak.
Therefor,e this vital energy
Cannot be halted by force,
Yet can be secured by inner power

Cannot be summoned by speech,
Yet can be welcomed by the awareness.
Reverently hold onto it and do not lose it:
This is called "developing inner power".
When inner power develops and wisdom emerges,
The myriad things will, to the last one, be grasped."

(Excerpt from 'Inward Training' (Nei-Yeh), a poem found in the Kuan Tzu, The Original Tao. translated by Harold D Roth, a text which the author thinks may predate the
Tao Te Ching.)

When is the Best Time to Practice, Life Is Healing Qigong?

Sunrise and sunset is the best time when the air is fresher. Any other time is also okay when there is a need to practice for healing purposes. It is best to practice on an empty stomach in the morning. Make sure the weather is not extreme. One should avoid cold, damp, scorching heat or drafty environments. These conditions can certainly make one ill and out of energetic balance. During inclement weather, it is advisable to practice indoor with plenty of fresh air. Avoid practicing during a thunderstorm or hurricane and after a big meal. Allow at least 1 hour after a meal before you practice. It is best to practice on an empty stomach.

Clothing

One should wear loose comfortable or warm clothing made of natural material such as wool, cotton or hemp. Shoes should be designed with a natural sole made from cotton, or leather. Avoid using rubber sneakers and

plastic soles which tends to block the flow of the earth's electromagnetic energy. Jewelry should be removed except for natural crystals such as quartz. Crystals can amplify one's energy if properly selected. Cell phones, watches, blue-tooth or any electronic device should also be removed to prevent electromagnetic field interference.

The Ideal Qigong Ecology

Practicing outdoors barefooted or with Chinese cotton slippers, moccasins are all ideal conditions for absorbing the earth's energy through the feet. You should always opt to practice on unpainted concrete, tile floors inside, grass, sand or dirt. Wood, carpet, linoleum surfaces tend to block or dampen the flow of the earth qi energy thus acting as an insulator. If you are indoors try practicing on a grounding pad. In depth Information on the use of grounding pads and how to obtain them can be found on the Earthing website at www.earthinginstitute.net

Almost any natural setting is ideal to practice. When you are indoors try to arrange your furniture to create better Feng Shui energy flow. Feng Shui is the art and science of arranging furniture and position objects in accordance with the principle of the 5 elements.

Chapter 3

Lifestyle Habits

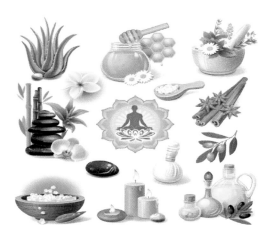

Nutrition is one of the 5 pillars of health necessary to sustain health and promote longevity. Life Is Healing Qigong emphasize eating only foods that are minimally processed without harmful food additives. There is no one diet for everyone because we are all energetically unique in terms of our constitution, energy expenditure and living environment. A Qigong practitioner should strive to eat according to the seasons and have a diverse diet.

For example, watermelon should not be eaten during the winter because its energy is damp and cold in nature. Everyone should try to avoid high fructose, corn syrup, MSG, canola oil, GMO foods, white flour and sugar, artificial sodas, red dye #40, yellow and blue food coloring as well. Smoking and alcohol should also be completely avoided especially when Qigong is used for healing purposes. As far as eating is concern, it is best to wait at least 1 hour before and after practicing. Water or warm tea can be taken in moderation at any time. Avoid cold or icy drinks prior to and after practice since cold energy can cause qi congestion.

Posture
The body should be relaxed, knees bowed, head lifted with elbows and shoulders lowered and chest sunken. Feet should be shoulder width apart. Meeting these standards is referred to as Song or Sung in Chinese or the relaxed natural state. One should also strive to have their tongue touch the upper palate of the mouth while doing Qigong postures and breathing. We

will go into more detail later about the position of the tongue during practice.

Breathing
One's breath should be deep, continuous, with even inhalation and exhalation through the nose. One's physical motions should follow the rhythm of the breath. Qigong emphasizes the use of the lower abdominal breathing known as natural breathing. This type of breathing should be done in place of upper chest shallow breathing.
Most breathing should be done through the nostrils except in cases of methods that require more explosive release of breath as seen in martial arts.

Other Attributes of Qigong

Grounding – Relates to developing an organic physical and mental connection with the earth by practicing stances. Grounding includes both static and moving base. Grounding leads one to experience inner security and peace. This form of Qi Gong is sometimes called Zhan Zhuang exercise which is associated with holding the tree, 3 circle standing or standing on the stakes to develop internal power.

Breathing -- extracting air or negatively charged ions is one of the primary goals of energy breathing. During qi breathing energy is drawn into the pores and bones. One can also breathe into the internal organs to promote better organ function via chi compression. Buddhist breathing is when the lower abdomen expands on inhalation), Taoist breathing is when the lower abdomen contracts on inhalation. The 5 healing sounds that correspond to the 5 Element Theory to purge the body of toxic qi are also part of medical and martial arts Qigong.

Connective Tissue Training Chan Su Chin Reeling Silk
This phase of training promotes joint flexibility, opening of energy meridians, and the purging of toxic qi and mineral deposits out of the tissue and joints. This phase of training prevents arthritis and weak bones.

4. Synchronizing Energy with Another. Sensitivity drills such as push hands, qi sao (sticky hands) and flowing chin- na teaches students how to manipulate qi in themselves and others. One can even eventually learn to harmonize their energy with the cosmos and Tao.

5. Guiding, Leading and Directing Qi – This energy is used to circulate in the body for purposes of healing. This healing energy can be extended outside the body for healing of others. It is now referred to as, External Qi Emission. This type of Qi Gong is sometimes referred to as Dao Yin/ Ying Qi Gong. Dao Yin exercises are characterized by continual slow, smooth movement guided by postural principles breath regulation and meditative attentiveness.

The "Inner School" of the martial arts, including Tai Ji and Bagua are best known for their fighting skills and principles as a reference for understanding and directing subtle forces.

(These various methods of Qigong will be discussed further in more detail in our future Qigong series.)

Yin / Yang

Yin is restorative in nature and is associated with nourishing the body with blood, DNA, hormones, and vital fluids such as synovial fluids for healthy joint movement. Yin is also a reflective, quiet, cooling, wet and meditative in nature. It personifies the feminine principle. Yang is the polar opposite of Yin. Its energy is expressive, explosive, extroverted, active, confronting and warming in nature. Yang personifies the masculine principle.

Polarity

There exists a polarity difference between a man and a woman. For a man, his head represents the Yin Pole while his groin represents the Yang Pole. It is just the opposite for a woman. A woman's head is her Yang Pole and her lower abdomen is her Yin Pole. This is why qi flows differently between the sexes and certain procedures like sealing in the qi upon conclusion of a qigong practice is done differently. The method of sealing in the qi after practice will be discussed later in this manual.

Chapter 4

Longevity, Martial Arts and The Athlete

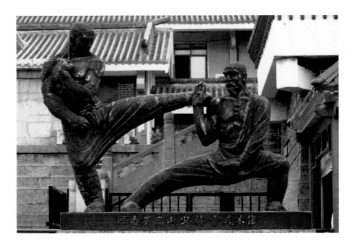

Shaolin Monks Practicing Kung-Fu

Qigong and Longevity

Our life span is determined by the quantity and quality of qi in our body. If the body is leaking qi due to injury, disease, poor diet or stress we tend to age faster. Repairing the body on a schedule basis can improve both the quality and quantity of our life force. Qigong can be quite a useful tool to facilitate this process. Our body should not be too yin or too yang in order to stay in balance. When we become too yang free radicals can create havoc throughout our bodies causing cellular deterioration and inflammation. Left unchecked these reactive responses can play a major role to accelerate our aging.

The Martial Artist and Athlete

In the west, we often admire the athletic physique and fitness level without really understanding that being an athlete is a competitive and sacrificing endeavor to achieve a specific goal. The athlete's goal is based upon specific skills to excel in a sporting event. This often requires overly strenuous training that often compromises their muscular skeletal system and cardio-vascular system.

Training in this manner is short term and requires huge expenditure of time, energy, money, sweat and a recovery period for the body to heal itself.

Such a way of life cannot be maintained on a long-term basis and eventually will lead to the decline of the athlete's health and fitness.

We must keep in mind that sports are for entertainment and not considered as a way of life. From a Qigong perspective, they often make the body too yang in terms of mental/emotional stress, overdevelopment of muscles and joint stresses. Much of these sacrifices are done to achieve a single goal of victory, a false sense of pride for some, over confidence and ego strokes. Modern society tends to place too much importance and overly reveres the athlete as the standard or ideal model for health.

Long term mortality studies clearly show that the athletes and allopathic doctors live no longer than the average non-athletic person. Health is not just athleticism nor the mere absence of disease. True long term health on having a sense of mental and emotional well-being, good qi flow and sound but balanced muscular/skeletal system free of inflammation. This is the truly goal of Qigong.

The foundation of martial arts is qigong. One should learn Qigong prior to learning martial arts. The foundation of martial arts which stresses breathing and focus is qigong. Both the athlete and martial artist should practice Qigong to stimulate the flow of qi the body and mind for more vigorous or tactical movement. The athlete should also consider using Qigong as a pre-workout warm up. Qigong can also be utilized as a wind down from intense movement and energy to help the body and mind recover from strenuous exercises. New research studies also show that Qigong recovery methods can facilitate the release of HGH or human growth hormones.

A recent study not yet published, coming out of California Poly Tech showed that athletes that spent 15 minutes a day doing Qigong exercises, were better rested, had lower cortisol, and significantly improved in their workouts, over others who do not engage in Qigong.

Chapter 5

The Major Energy Centers in the Body

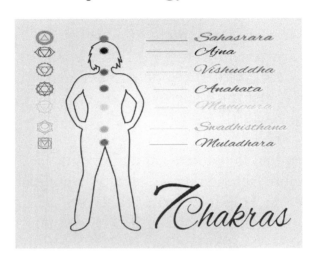

What are the 6 Major Energy Vortices in the Body?

Yong Quang - (bubbling springs) is located on the bottom of the foot at the metatarsal.
Hui Yin – is located between the anus and the genital area call the perineum.
Dan Tien- (sea of qi) is located 3 inches below the umbilicus. It is the storage battery or reservoir for the body's energy.
Ming Men – is located at the tail bone.
Huao Tio – is in the hip area near the sciatic region.
Bai Hui – is located at the crown of the head in the area of the fontanel
Yin Ta i- (third eye) is located in the area between the eyes.
Lao Gong – is located on the center of the palms known as the hand chakra.

What Are the 3 Dan Tiens?

Lower Dan Tien, about four fingers widths below your navel, is where you store jing or your kidney essence.
Middle Dan Tien, in the area of your heart, is where you gather your qi or vitality.

Upper Dan Tien or your third eye between the eyebrows inside your forehead, is where you gather your Shen or spiritual energy.
In Chinese medicine the heart is referred to as the emperor of the body and the second brain. It circulates not only blood but also your qi. An old Chinese saying states that when your heart is happy, the rest of your organs will be happy too. Together, your Jing, Qi and Shen are known as the 3 treasures, When your three treasures are balanced, you experience radiant health and longevity.

The 3 Major Dan Tiens

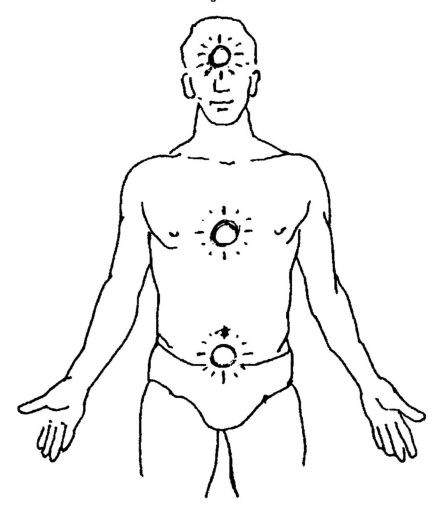

The 3 Dan Tiens (energy centers) are located on the Ta Ji Pole or Chong Mei Meridian. This meridian runs up the center of the body from the perineum to the crown of the head supplying energy to all the other meridians. The Dan Tien is sometimes referred to as the lower, middle and upper or burners or Jiao in Chinese. These areas correspond to the lower

middle and upper regions of the body and their anatomical and visceral functions.

The circulation of qi up the middle back (Governor Vessel) and down the front torso (Conception Vessel) is called the Microcosmic Circulation. When learning Qigong, it is very important to understand and practice this form of qi circulation before proceeding to more advanced form of energy manipulation such as the Macrocosmic Circulation of Qi. A more detail explanation of both forms of qi circulation will be discussed in our future series.

What are Energy Meridians?

Meridians are known as the energy mapped pathways of qi or vital energy to flow into and out of the body. Each pathway is named and usually corresponds to a yin or yang organ. An example of this relationship is the kidney/bladder meridian. There are 6 yin and 6 yang organs in addition to 8 Psychic Channels that are not associated with any internal organs. The two main Psychic Channels are referred to as the Conception Vessel (Ren Mai) or CV and the Governor Vessel (Du Mai) or GV which is located up the middle of the back. Meridians are very much like nerve pathways. The energy in the meridians are either balanced, deficient or in excess.

The Tai Qi Pole also known as Kundalini and Chong Mai Vessel should be the focus point for most Qigong practitioner. This meridian runs up the middle of the body and is not associated with any body part or organ. It is referred to as in Chines medicine as one of the 8 Psychic Channels or Strange Flows. Ren Mai and Du Mai are also psychic channels. These channels draw energy directly into the body for emergency or for some focus intent.

(See Illustration on the next page)

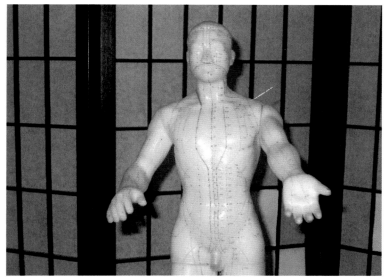

The Ren/Conception Yin Vessel runs up the center axis of the front upper torso of the body.

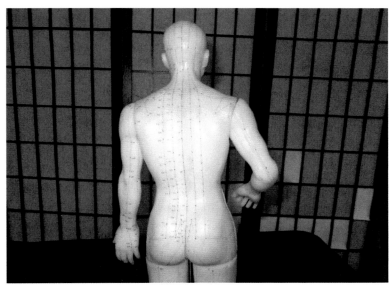

Th Du/Governor Yang Vessel runs up the center axis of the rear upper torso of the body.

These two vessels are part of the what is known as the Micro- Cosmic Orbit of Qi Circulation. These two vessels alone are responsible for many miraculous healing within the body.
They are not associated with any specific organs but have a profound influence in relationship how energy flows in and out of each organ.

Chapter 6

The 4 Basic States of Energetic Health

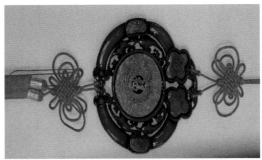
Jade Chakra

Energy States

1. Deficient,
2. Excess,
3. Balanced/Flowing and
4. Block Stagnant Flow

Simple Explanation of the Basic 4 States of Energy

Excess Qi:

If you put too much energy into a weak vessel it will overload, short circuit and cause weakness. An example of this is overtraining and stress.

Deficient Qi:

If a person does not have enough energy to ignite wood a camp fire will never combust. There will be no warmth or comfort to experience.

Block or Stagnant Qi:

If energy is blocked or stuck there will be no flow of current to nourish the body. This condition will usually cause pain or discomfort. An example, If a water hose is bent it will build pressure at the point of the bend causing a bulge. The water pressure will eventually build to the point of a rupture. The intended destination of the water to irrigate the flower or lawn will be disrupted.

Flowing Balance:

Vital energy flows naturally and nourishes all body and mind functions to create a sense of well- being and radiant health. A simple example would be a recycling water fountain pump. In this case, water energy flows and recycles itself naturally without a spill.

Element Theory

The 5 Element Theory is closely connected with the 5 yin/yang internal organ system. The 5 elements are fire, water, earth, wood and metal (sometimes referred to as air). The 5 Element Theory also explains and illustrates the correlation between the 5 elemental energies and their emotional correspondence.

The kidneys are associated with the Water element. The Spleen is considered to be Earth. The heart is connected to Fire. Liver is of the Wood element. Lungs are associated with the Metal Element.
A Qigong practitioner should be able to relate specific Qigong exercises to specific health problems. This is done by over-standing how Qigong exercises are connected to the 5element principle and energy organ system. The 5 Element Theory in addition to Qigong encompasses the use of herbs, acupuncture, massage and essential oils which can be used to make liniments or taken internally under guidance.

Out of all the 5 organs, the kidneys are considered the most important according to Chinese medicine and health. They are the foundational energy that determines the quantity and quality of our life span. The kidneys represent our ultimate source of jing (essence) and serves as a deeper reservoir of our primal qi.

The areas that are impacted by the kidney qi are hearing, bone marrow, teeth, sexual energy and reproduction, immunity. athletic ability and the body's ability to heal itself can be linked to the kidneys. If you are limited by time and are trying to decide which posture to practice, make the decision to always target your kidney energy.

The Table of Correspondences & The Five Elements

Element	Wood	Fire	Earth	Metal	Water
Season	Spring	Summer	Late Summer	Autumn	Winter
Yang Organ	Gall Bladder	Small Intestine Triple Heater	Stomach	Colon	Bladder
Yin Organ	Liver	Heart Pericardium	Spleen	Lungs	Kidneys
Emotion	Anger	Joy	Sympathy	Grief	Fear
Color	Green	Red	Yellow	White	Blue
Sound	Shouting	Laughing	Singing	Weeping	Groaning
Taste	Sour	Bitter	Sweet	Pungent	Salty
Smell	Rancid	Scorched	Fragrant	Rotten	Putrid
Opening	Eyes	Tongue	Mouth	Nose	Ears
Tissue	Tendons	Blood Vessels	Flesh	Skin and Hair	Bones
Climate	Wind	Heat	Damp	Dry	Cold
Process	Birth	Growth	Transformation	Harvest	Storage
Direction	East	South	Centre	Wind	North

Chapter 7

Qigong and Essential Oils Connection

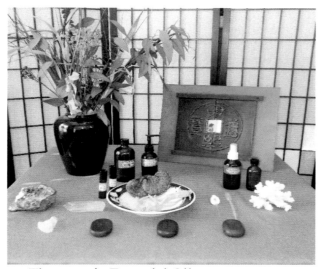
Therapeutic Essential Oils

Ever wondered if the therapeutic benefits of essential oils and Qigong are a good combination? Yes, very much so.

What Are Essential Oils?

Essential oils are extracted directly from the bark, flower, fruit, leaf, seed or root of a plant or tree. Just one drop can have powerful health benefits. Essential oils are created through the process of steam distillation which separates the oil and water. These oils are often more powerful than the herbs because they contain volatile compounds in a more concentrated form. The essence of the body is blood. The essence of a plant or herb is stored in its oil. These natural oils in plants protect the plant from insects, shield the plant from a harsh environment and help them adapt to their surroundings. By using essential oils, you are harnessing the protective and potent healing powers of a botanical.

Essential oils are truly the most potent form of plant based medicine. Their power to heal and cure disease is so effective that by using essential oils many people can avoid the need to use of synthetic drugs or have risky types of invasive surgeries. The essential oils can also be used to help one recover from an intense workout or fatigue. Essential oils are composed of very small molecules that can penetrate your cells especially when rubbed on the feet. Some of the compounds in essential oils can even cross the blood-brain barrier.

  Essential oils differ from fatty oils like those in vegetables or nuts. Cooking oils are made up of large molecules that cannot penetrate your cells. They are not as therapeutic in the same manner when used topically. In contrast, essential oils can be used topically, inhaled using a nebulizer, taken internally (with the help of a trained professional) and used in many personal care products.

(The Kings Medicine Cabinet by Dr. Josh Axe,
The Essential Life a Guide to Living The Wellness Lifestyle 2nd Edition)

The History Essential Oils and Ancient Egypt

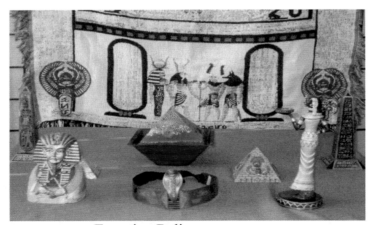

Egyptian Relics

The Egyptians are usually credited as the true founders of aromatherapy dating back to 4500B.C. The Egyptians were masters in using essential oils and other aromatics for healing emotions and negative energy. Historical records describe how one of the founders of the "pharaonic" medicine was the architect, Imhotep. Imhotep lived during the reign of King Djoser (2630-

2611BC) and was the architect of the step pyramid at Saqquara, the first pyramid ever built in Egypt.

Imhotep was worshipped as a god and healer from approximately 2850 B.C to 525 B.C. He was a known scribe, chief lector, priest, astronomer and magician. (Medicine and magic were used together).

Imhotep became the second king of Egypt's third dynasty, who was later worshiped as the god of medicine in Egypt and in Greece.
He was identified with the Greek god of medicine Asclepius.
 Imhotep became the Grand Vizier of *King Djoser*. ¨
 He was also a poet and philosopher.
He was considered by many to be the real Father of Medicine – where he ushered in the use of oils, herbs, and aromatic plants for medicinal purposes.

Hieroglyphs on the walls of the Egyptian temples depict the blending of oils and describe hundreds of oil recipes.
Ancient Egyptian papyrus found in the temple of Edfu, contained formulations to make medicines and perfumes used by the alchemists and high priests.
They were also known to design personal perfumes to elicit various emotions and inspire thoughts.
In 1922, when King Tut's tomb was opened, 350 liters of oils were discovered in alabaster jars. Plant waxes had solidified into a thickened residue around the inside of the container openings, leaving the liquefied oil in excellent condition.

According to ancient Egyptian hieroglyphs, priests and alchemists were using essential oils thousands of years ago, to heal the sick and used for many spiritual rituals. The Egyptians believed that the sense of smell and the ability to detect odors was the most important of the sensory abilities. Why? Because they knew that the inhalation of essential oils can increase one's frequency, affect the pineal gland- the divine connector to enlightenment. These oils served as the catalyst to transformation of negative energy into higher spiritual powers. Imhotep was worshipped as a god and healer from approximately 2850 B.C to 525 B.C. He was a known scribe, chief lector, priest, astronomer and magician. Medicine and magic were often used together to heal the incurables.

References:
http://www.raindropeducation.com/id74.html

How Can I Use Essential Oils for Qigong?

The answer is very simple. When practicing Qigong indoors during cold weather, essential oils can be used to promote deep breathing, focus and positive mood. Oils such as peppermint and citrus are very energizing in contrast to oils such as frankincense and myrrh which tend to promote relaxation and cleansing. Many of these oils can be very helpful when doing both Qigong meditation and postures.

According to Traditional Chinese Medicine essential oils can be classified as Yin or yang or more yin and less yang or more yang and less yin. Many of these oils can be linked to one or more of the 5 elements, fire, earth, water, metal(air) and wood. Let us briefly examine a few oils to help us understand this relationship.

Cinnamon Oil is a yang oil due to its warming nature and is linked to the element fire and associated with increasing circulation of blood and improving digestion which are associated with the lower and middle burner of the body.

Spearmint Oil is more yin in nature and has a cooling effect on the body and can be associated with the elements water and metal (air) used to improve breathing functions in the body. Eucalyptus Oil could also easily fit in this same category as well. These are only few examples of how oils can be classified under the 5 Element Theory of medicinal usage.

Combining the use of herbs and essential oils with your Qigong practice can truly enhance healing and a more powerful synergistic effect than using them separately. If you are experiencing low back pain due to muscle strain try rubbing some cinnamon oil diluted with a carrier oil (fractionated coconut oil, jojoba, olive or grapeseed oil) prior to doing the Kidney Qigong posture. The combination of the oil and the posture can significantly reduce recovery time. I personally use essential daily both internally and topically when I practice Qigong.

A note of caution, some essential oils are too potent like as peppermint to be applied directly to the skin and need to be diluted with a carrier oil such as coconut oil. Taking essential oils internally should be done under the guidance of an experienced aromatherapist due to their potency.

The Life Is Healing School of Qigong highly recommends that students of martial arts, qigong, foot reflexology or just about everyone interested in improving their health may good use of tonic herbs and aromatic essential oils.

For more detailed information about the selection, type and best grades of essential oils to buy please visit our website at:

mydoterra.com/lifeishealing

Chapter 8

Qigong Energy Supplements

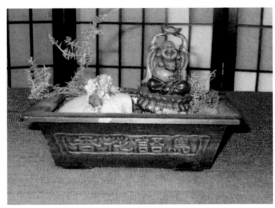

The Happy Healthy Buddha

Tonic Herbs

There are many herbal formulas and individual herbs that are beneficial to Qigong practitioners. Out of these many herbs we recommend using the premier tonic herbs such as Schizandra Berries, Red Reshi, Cordyceps, Gogi Berries and Astragulus according to the 5 Element Principle. For example, Hou shou Wu is often known as the primary kidney/liver herb because it energetically influences the flow of qi in both kidney/liver meridians. Cordyceps, one of my favorite for cycling is often used to tonify the lung function and improve endurance. All of these premier herbs above tend to strengthen the body's immune system, builds physical strength, calm the mind and spirit. Many Taoist monks also use these herbs to enhance the sexual energy of the body that is associated with kidney yang qi. and reproductive system.

 When consuming tonic herbs one needs not be concern with cycling on and off days. The effect of daily consumption is cumulative and usually peaks over the course of 90-100 days for full cellular saturation. These herbs can be taken for life as they also build Jing, Qi, and Shen or the 3 treasures as described earlier in this manual.

Comparing Qigong to a Car Engine

Qigong is a dual energy mechanism very much similar to a car engine. It is both electrical and combustible in nature.

Kidneys are very much like a battery with water and dissolved electrolytes which provide electrical energy. It is the primary energy source of the body. Its emotional connection is fear flight or fight.

Spleen represents food or gasoline to produce energy in the form of blood, It is emotionally connected to worry and over planning or thinking

Heart is the pump and piston of the body. It provides and heat and drives the blood/qi. Its emotional connection is to joy or hatred.

Liver circulates blood to all parts of the body and releases energy when needed for extra acceleration much like a fuel injection or fuel pump in a car. It is associated with the emotion anger or irritability.

Lungs provide oxygen for ignition (oxidizer) to help regulate the demand for more changing needs. Its emotional component is grief and sadness.

Bio-Electric Magnet

The reason that Chi is the most important single factor in health is because your entire body is essentially a large bio-electric magnet. Without these magnetic fields, our cellular activity would cease to function. Life could not occur. Our trillions of cells have an electromagnetic field (EM) and that keeps each cell alive. The stronger the EM field, the stronger each cell is and the greater is it resilience and resistance to degeneration.

This is one of the main reasons that Qigong should be practice on earth conducting surfaces barefoot or with natural conducting shoes such as cotton sole or leather or moccasin shoes whenever possible. The earth's magnetic field is measured in gauss. The magnetic field of the earth is weakening. At present, the earth's field strength is only 0.5 gauss as compared to the past when the field was greater than 1. I recommend the use of magnetic insoles place into your shoes or standing on top of magnetics with a field strength range of 3,000 -5000 gauss for maximum penetration into the feet and meridians. Magnetic grounding pads can be purchased and used as a mattress for sitting meditation or indoor training during those times when the weather is too severe for outdoor training.

Dr. Andrew Weil cites several studies that suggest magnets have much to offer in the area of pain relief:

• A 1997 study at Baylor College of Medicine in Houston showed that 76 percent of patients treated with magnets for severe joint and muscle pain due to post-polio syndrome reported less pain compared to only 19 percent of those who received placebos.

• University of Virginia researchers said participants reported clinically meaningful improvements when using magnet therapy to reduce the intensity of pain from fibromyalgia.

• A University of Tennessee study showed that 60 percent of women with pelvic pain reported improvements after three weeks of magnet therapy compared to 33 percent of those treated with placebos.

How to Evaluate the Effectiveness of Your Qigong Training

1. One must first be able to understand which organ exercise can cause the desired effect on well- being and balance.

2. Keeping track of progress and targeting those areas or symptoms of concern is paramount to successful healing.

3. Other methods for supporting and influencing qi should be explored such as diet and herbs previously to create a balance of yin and yang.

4. Much of the benefits derived from Qigong practice are usually cumulative over the course of 90 to 100 days.

In summary, one should be able to relate specific Qigong exercises to specific health problems. This is done by over-standing how Qigong exercises are related to the 5 Element Principle and energy organ systems.

Benefits Associated with Regular Qigong Practice

Vitality   Improved mental performance
Alertness   increased libido and sexual energy
Endurance   enhanced memory
Facilitated healing   better relaxation and sleep
Emotional stability   reduced symptoms of aging
Improved flexibility   emotional calm and positive outlook
Higher pain tolerance   stronger immune system
Strengthen joints and balance   muscular skeletal connective tissue

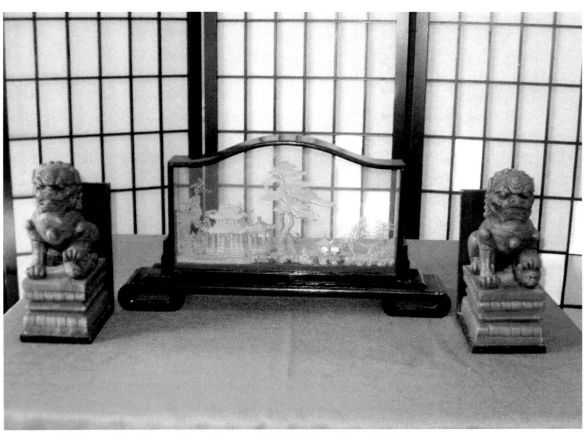

Chinese Fu Dogs, Guardians of Forbidden Knowledge

Chapter 9

The Story of Li Ching-Yuen?

The story everyone should know about the Qigong master Li Ching-Yuen is quite incredible.

Go to this website to view a clear picture of him.
http://plantcures.com/Lichingyun.html

Li Ching-Yuen was born in 1678 A.D. and died in 1928 at the age of 250 years old. Li was a herbalist, and Chi Kung Master and lived in the mountains most of his life. After his death, General Yang investigated Li's background to verify his true age and determined Li was telling the truth. He authored a report "A Factual Account of the 256-Year-Old Good Luck Man."

Li Ching-Yuen was born in 1678, during the seventeenth year of the Manchu Emperor Kang Shi's Reign. He left home at an early age and traveled around southern China with a group of itinerant herb traders, from whom he learned the basics of herbalism.
Subsequently, Li had the good fortune to meet several highly accomplished Taoist masters, who taught him internal alchemy and chi-gung and showed him how to utilize diet and herbal supplements for health and longevity. Master Li was not a celibate. Over the course of his long life he married 14 times, and by the time of his death in 1933, he counted almost 200 living descendants within his extended family.

After his death, modern scholars confirmed his identity, traced his life all the way back to the year of his birth, and conclusively verified his lifespan. Master Lee's life demonstrates how well Taoist longevity techniques work when properly practiced. Master Li continued to take long hikes in the mountains until the final years of his life; he remained sexually active for over two centuries, never became senile and died with all of his own teeth and most of his hair.
Master Li's Diet, occasionally consist of small bits of meat. He was not a strict vegetarian. He limited the intake of grains and root vegetables. His daily diet consisted mostly of fruit lightly steamed vegetables.

Master Li's Herbal Supplements, Ginseng, Gotu Kola, Polygonum Multiflorum, and Garlic. There was also a recipe for a Spring Tonic concocted by Master Li.
(The Complete Book of Chinese Health and Healing by Daniel Reid")

Although Master Li is an extreme example of what Qigong, diet and herbs can do to enhance longevity one should not take his story as fictional.

The following gives an unabridged compilation of all the benefits associated with the practice of Qigong. Many of these benefits have been documented by the Chinese government and their Medical Qigong Universities.
Qigong increases neural pathways created in both hemispheres of the brain, resulting in what is known as "whole-brain functioning," which enhances creativity, intuition, and increased learning ability. Qigong is not a religious practice, but it can be a spiritual path. It gives a sense of oneness with the universe. enlightenment, The Buddha and the Tao.

Remember all Qi gong exercises must have 3 attributes to be therapeutic and complete:
Posture
Breathing
Focus creative visualization

Qigong is a multi-purpose healing modality depending upon the need. Think of it as a tool box with many functions. Qigong has varying applications. Some of them are simple and generic, while others are so complicated that you need specialized instruction from someone who is trained and experienced. It is as important to select the right tool and understand the method of use.

Qigong Multiple Applications

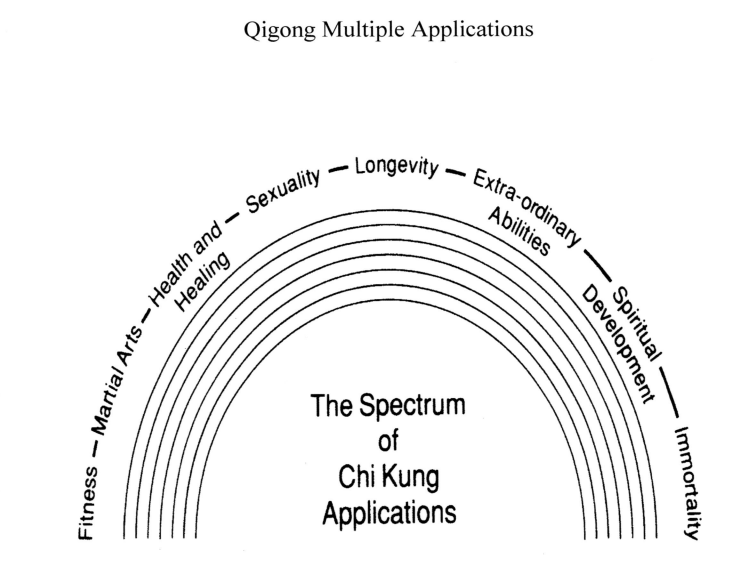

Fitness — Martial Arts — Health and Healing — Sexuality — Longevity — Extra-ordinary Abilities — Spiritual Development — Immortality

The Spectrum
of
Chi Kung
Applications

Chapter 10

13 Basics Harmonies and Alignments of the Body

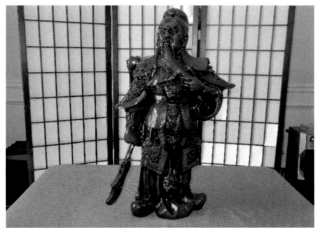

General Kwan Yu, guardian patriot

Learning to apply progressive relaxation both internally and externally is a must. Qigong starts with the Wu Qi concept of emptying the mind and feeling the center of the body, the lower Dan Tien, while achieving a rooted sensation in the legs. When conducting postures a student should adhere to the following key points:

1. Keep elbows relax and sunken.
2. Release the chest and sink the shoulders.
3. Suspend head upward while elongating your spine downward.
4. Slighting tuck buttocks inward and contract the anus gently
5. Sit on your hips with a erect spine.
6. Float your wrist and open the hands to express the fingers like reeling silk (Chan Si Jing), while your eyes follow your hands directly or indirectly.
7. Shift weight from the ball of the foot to the heels.
8. Breathe through the nose deeply and slowly using abdominal breathing.
9. Place tongue in the upper palette behind the teeth.
10. Mentally project your body root several feet below the surface of the earth while gripping and scrunching your toes to the ground like a tiger.
11. Apply an abduction force to the leg like squeezing a ball between them or reverse abduction force by pushing the legs and feet outward.

12. Keep knees over the instep when bent to avoid knee strain.
13. All movement should be in coordination with the breath.

I know this is a lot to take in all at once. You should strive to work on a few pointers at a time and be mindful on an ongoing basis of the others. You can also use these pointers to gauge your progress and make self -correction when you feel out of alignment or your flow is off. Remember energy must also have an anatomy to flow properly. Form follows function.

Chapter 11

Qigong Warm-Ups

Before beginning your Qigong warm-up stand in a relaxed manner and circle your neck 10 times to the left and right side in a gentle manner.
Then proceed to do hip circles 10 times on both side of your body

1. **Rotary Breathing -** Our Qigong starts with breathing and gentle movement of the spine. Place your hands alongside of your chest as if holding a large ball. Inhale and exhale deeply through the nose while circling your hands forward in a rotary type motion coordinated with the breath. Retain the breath after inhalations for several seconds between cycles. Repeat this movement 5-10 times.

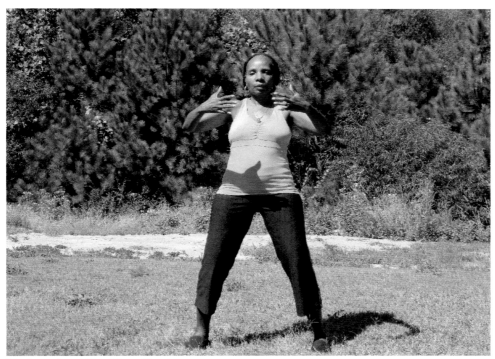

Embracing The Tree Posture

2. **Prisoner of War Breathing Posture**   In the next sequence you will raise your hands up along your sides and up until your hands are behind your head like a prisoner of war. Stretch out your chest and scapula area. Inhale in this position retaining your breath for several seconds then lower your

arms to the side while exhaling through the nose. Repeat this movement 5-10 times to charge your body with qi.

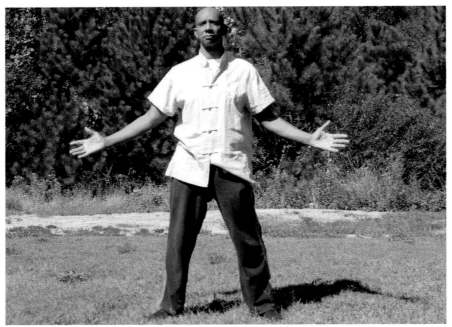

Raise hands up along the side of the body.

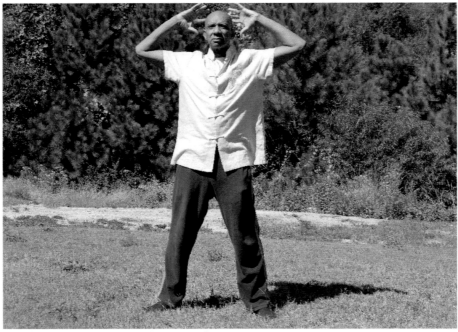

Prisoner of War Posture

Breathe in deep 5 -10 times with breath retention with your hands behind your head. Then lower your hands back along the side body.

3. **Dragon Twists Body** - Turn your body side to side while allowing your arms to swing up against the front and back of the body. On each swing one of your palms should lightly tap your kidney while the other impacts your spleen or liver on the front side of your abdomen. These motions should be done in a smooth rhythmic manner. Your head, shoulder and hip should be aligned on the same frontal axis.

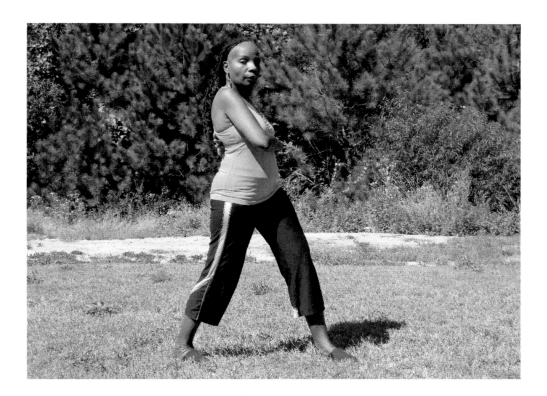

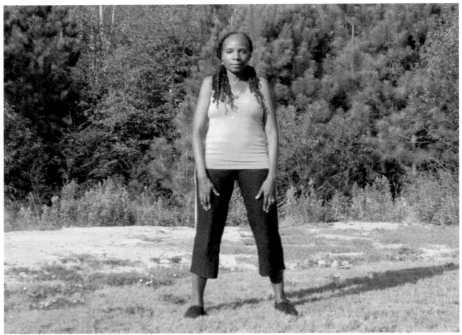

Start in the Wu Qi posture staring forward

4. Raising the Arms and Sweeping the Earth

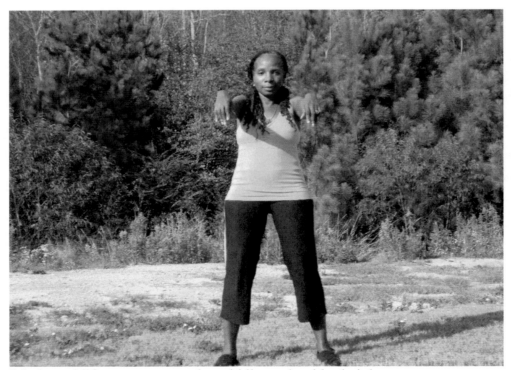

Inhale and lift your arms up the middle to shoulder height.

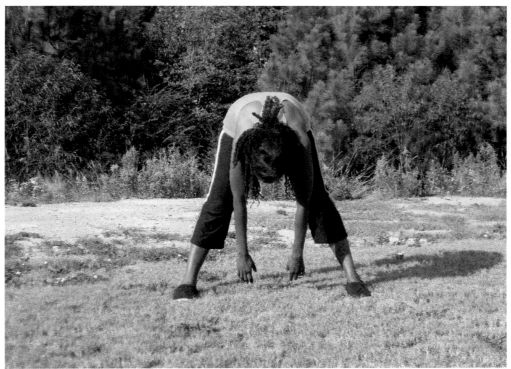

Exhale and lower your arms to stretch down to the earth without bending your knees

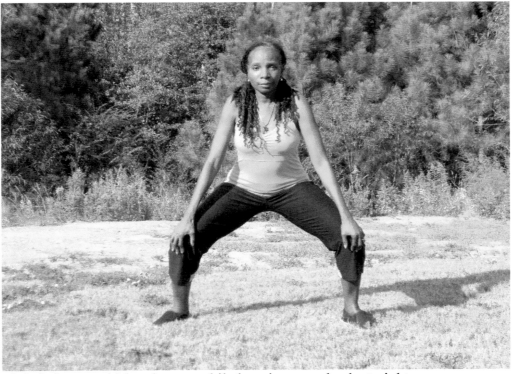

Inhale into a mid-level squat while keeping your back straight.

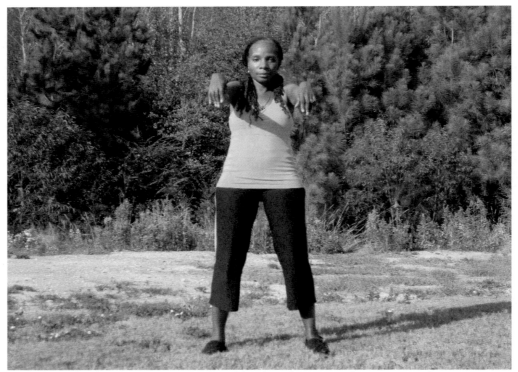

Exhale and raise your arms to shoulder level to complete one cycle.

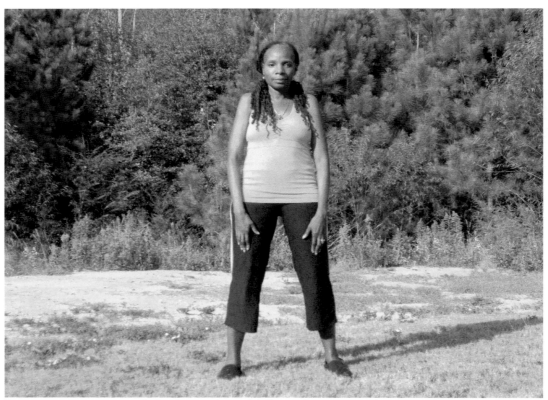

Lower your arms straight down the middle and return to the Wu Qi Posture.

Congratulation! You have completed your warm- ups.

You are now ready to begin the 5 Taoist Yin Organ Qigong Exercise
If you are still confused as how to do the energy warm ups or 5 Organ
Qigong sequences properly, please refer to our guided DVD for help.

For steady progress remember to always do the following:

1. Stay mentally calm, physically relax and focused.
2. Coordinate your breathing with your movement.
3. Breathe slow and deep inhaling and exhaling through the nose.
4. Try to feel for the sensation of qi flow through your torso and limbs.
5. Avoid practicing when emotionally upset or fatigued.
6. Keep the tip of your tongue connected to the top of your mouth.

What does Qi Feel Like?

The Sensation of Qi is felt when you move your limbs as you were reeling
silk. These movements should be light, flowing and delicate to increase your
ability to feel qi. The sensation of qi varies from person to person. It can
sometimes be described as a tingling feeling, expanding feeling, full or
heavy sensation, heat or warm flow of fluids through your body. When you
sense something pleasant happening to you, it is more than likely your qi at
work.

The Importance of the Tongue Position

Many Qigong practitioner fail to reap the full benefit of their practice by not
understanding the role of the tongue switch and its placement. The tongue is
the connecting switch for the qi to flow through the meridians. The lower
and upper areas of the mouth or palate are designated zones that are specific
to the flow of qi completing an orbit or circuit. Each of the 5 Yin Organs
have their own position. Only the tip of the tongue is used to complete the
proper placement.

The 5 Yin Organs Tongue Positions

Lung Point // located on the center upper palate behind the upper row of teeth on the gum line

Liver Point // located on the middle of the upper palate perpendicular to the jaw line

Kidney Point // the tongue must be curled to the back of the upper palate

Heart Point // located between the lung point and the Liver area on the upper palate.

Spleen Point // the tip of the tongue is placed on the center gum line behind bottom row of the teeth

One should maintain the position of the tongue while breathing from the stomach and moving in coordination with the breath for each sequence while applying abduction and outer flexion of the legs.

Adhering to these guidelines will enable a practitioner to achieve maximum benefits *

Chapter 12

Pulling up Earth and Pulling Down Heaven

Okay Let's Get Started!

[Opening Movement]

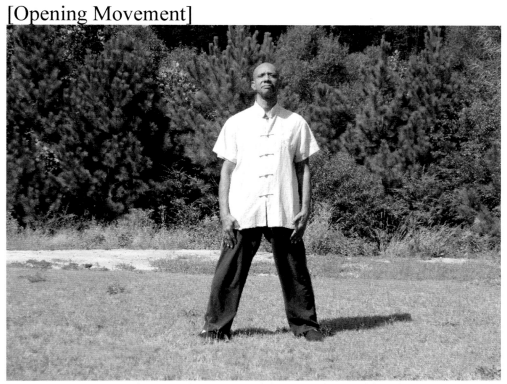

Start with the Wu Qi Neutral Posture with normal breathing

Important Note:

When drawing the qi upward, lifting your arms or merging your hands together gently squeeze your abductor or inner thigh muscles and feet inward. When pushing out to the sides or lowering your arms you should push down and outward with your legs. Remember, these motions should be done while gently contracting your anus muscle. All movement should be coordinated with your breathing while keeping your muscles relax and supple. Your breath should be quiet and deep. Keep your mind focused on your breath and movement

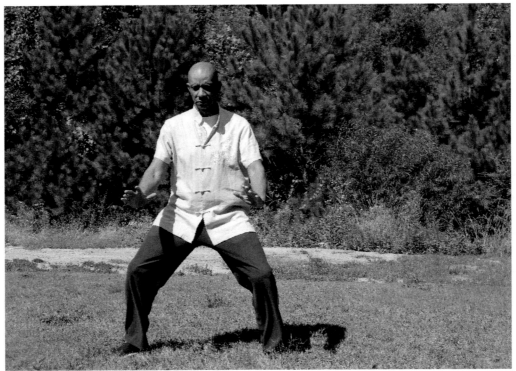

Inhale deeply and form your hands as lifting up a large ball from the ground then exhale and push the energy ball back into the ground

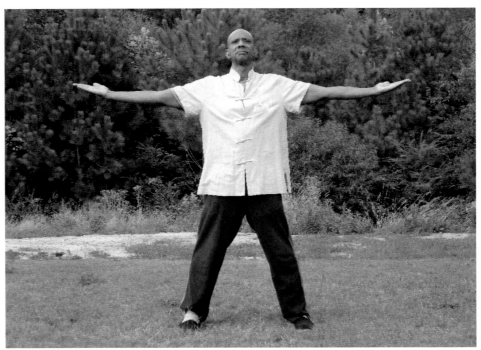

Inhale and begin to raise hands upward slowly along the sides of body.

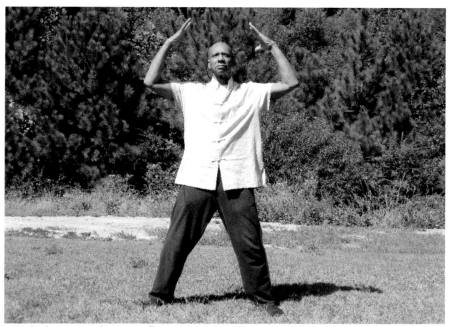

Exhale, stretch your fingers and pull energy from heaven down into the crown of the head and channel this energy down through the chest and lower torso.

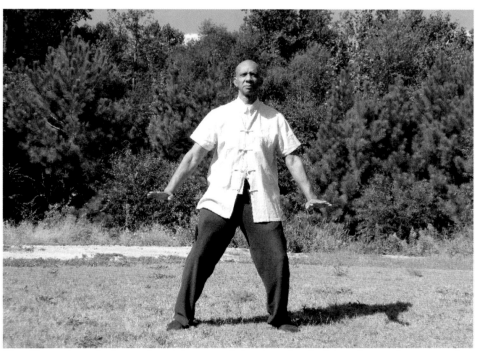

Continue to exhale and guide your intent and mind to channel energy down into the legs.

The purpose of this movement is to consciously bring the cosmic energy and earth qi into the body through the Tai Qi Pole central axis storing it into the lower Dan Tien located 4 fingers located below the navel or umbilicus. The term cosmic energy refers to the lunar, solar and cosmic high energy emission from interstellar space that inundates the earth every second. The Tai Qi Pole Axis is also known as the Kundalini or Chong Mei Energy Channel that runs from the lower Dan Tien up the middle of the body to the fontanel or crown chakra of the head.

While standing lower your body to a half squat with an erect spine aligned; then reach your arms down as if grabbing a large beach ball sitting on the ground in front of you. When doing so perform a reverse abdominal breathing pattern drawing your abdomen in on inhalation and outward on exhalation. This is known as the Taoist Breath. Lift the imaginary energy ball up to your abdomen drawing it into your body and then lower it back down on the ground. Now reach your hands up on your sides as if you are lifting a huge beach ball up above your head. Once above your head proceed to pull this ball down through the center of your head and body progressing to press the ball downward to the ground. (For further assistance see our DVD)

Taoist 5 Organ Medical Qigong Application

Please note that the Taoist 5 Yin Organs Qigong is a tonifying and balancing organ exercise used to improve a chronically weak organ function or when there is a condition of excess or deficient qi. A good example of this would be a person who has chronic low back pain due to weak kidney qi versus a person who has low back pain due to muscle strain caused by improper lifting. Low chronic back pain caused by weak kidney qi can be ameliorated by the 5 organs kidney posture whereas, low back strain needs to be treated differently. This is reason why this type of Qigong is classified as a medical qigong.

The 5 Yin Organs System of Qigong is best used as a preventative measure to avoid imbalances that could lead to illness. Do not practice the Taoist 5 Yin Organs Qigong when you are physically or mentally fatigue, experiencing chronic pain or suffering from a recent traumatic injury, soft tissue trauma or acute inflammation. In our future series, we will discuss measures to take to help alleviate those types of conditions.

Contra-Indications
The 5 Yin Organs exercises should not be performed if you have a bacterial or viral infection, broken bones, are on your menses or pregnant. There are no restrictions however for the lung posture since we are always breathing.

Chapter 13

The 5 Organ Taoist Qigong Postures

The beginning sequence starts with the lung activation posture as seen below. These postures can be practiced standing or seated if needed. One should also smile gently into the organs and envision a specific color of bright light filling it up. The only exceptions are for the liver and turtle postures which you do not smile when performing.

Lung/Large Intestine
Activate with/ white light, smile into the organ tongue is placed behind upper teeth.

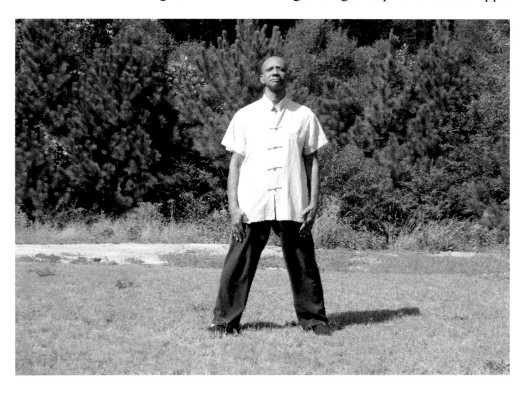

Start this posture in the Wu Qi relax neutral posture with normal breathing.

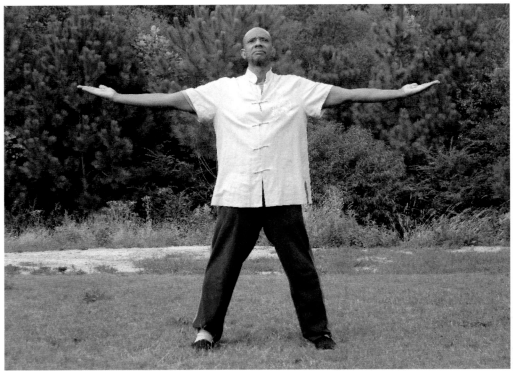

Raise arms out to your sides with palms facing up while inhaling.

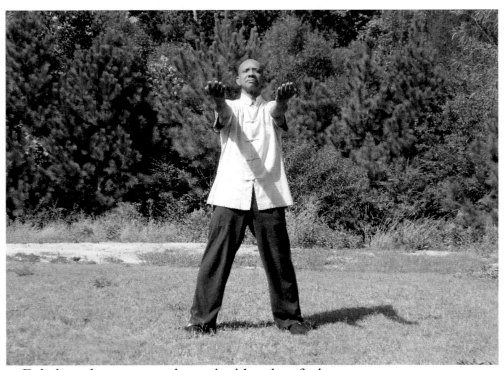

Exhale and rotate arms inward with palms facing up.

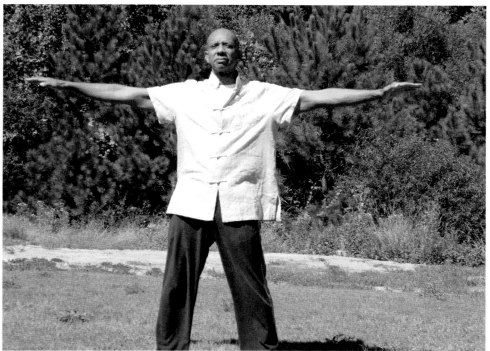

Inhale and smile into your lungs and envision bright white light filling them up while rotating your arms out to the side with palms down.

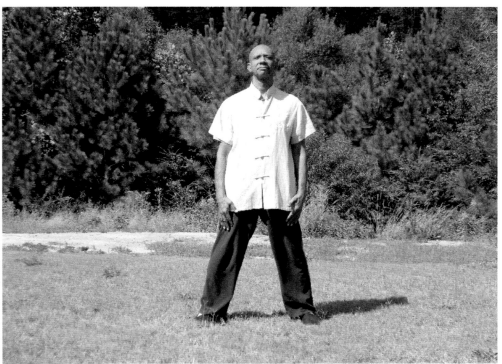

End sequence by returning your arms back to the center with palms down lowering them to your sides in the Wu Qi Posture.

Lungs/ Instructions

1. Stand in the Wu Qi opening stance.
2. Inhale, lift and rotate your arms and palms upward from your sides to shoulder level.
3. Move your arms inward with both palms facing up towards the center of your chest. Repeat movements ten times.
4. End the sequence by returning your arms back to center and rotate your palms downward then lower your arms.

Association

Organ – Lungs/Large Intestine
Elements – Metal
Season – Fall or Autumn
Color – White
Emotion – Sadness or inspiration

Benefits

This posture helps to improve the function of the lungs, nasal congestion, skin, depression, colds, shallow breathing and issues with grief, sadness or depression. Practice this posture more often during the fall season to help maintain balance, increase your Wei Qi (resistance) and prevent respiratory discomforts or seasonal affective depression (SAD) or mood swings.

Liver/Gallbladder

Activate with /green light, look bold/tongue touches the upper palate just before the middle point.

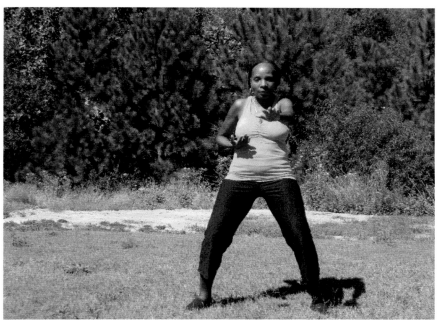

Sit in a horse stance, stare fiercely and thrust your left hand forward alternating with your right hand Imagine breaking a board with your palms. Your hips should swivel with each palm thrust. Can be done with palms facing downward or erected.

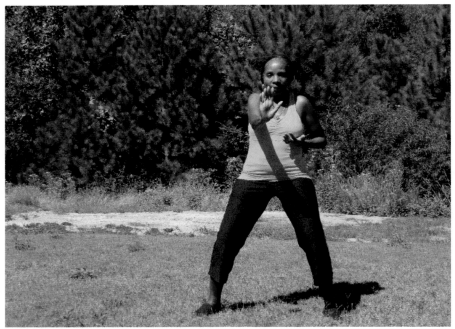
Do the same with your opposite hand.

Liver Activation Instructions

1. Sit in a frontal like horse stance
2. Twist your hips while shooting out your palm with a sharp eye focus
3. Do the same on with your other palm
4. Inhale envision green bright light as you withdraw your hands, exhale as you thrust them forward.
5. Perform this sequence a total of 10-20 times

Association

Organ – Liver/Gallbladder
Elements – Wood
Season - Spring
Color – Green
Emotion – Anger Release

Benefits

   This posture helps to improve the function of the eyes, tendons muscles, ligaments and anger issues. Practice the liver posture more often during the spring seasons to help maintain balance and encourage detoxification of the body.

Chapter 14

Opening the Kidneys

Kidney/Bladder
Activate with royal blue, smile into the organ/curl tongue to the rear of the upper palate.

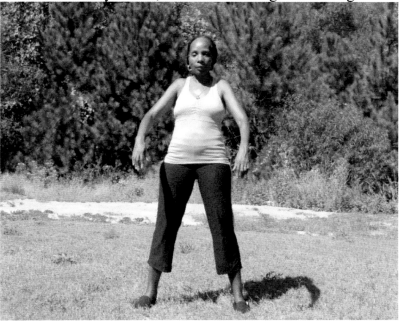

Begin by standing in a focused relax manner with normal breathing.

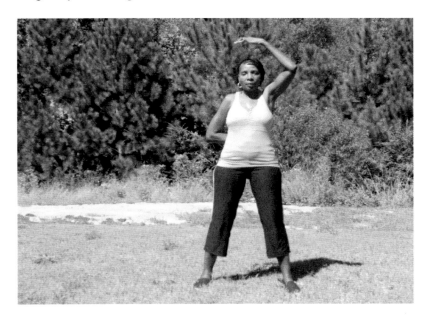

Inhale deep royal blue light and place the back of your rear right hand   on your left kidney.

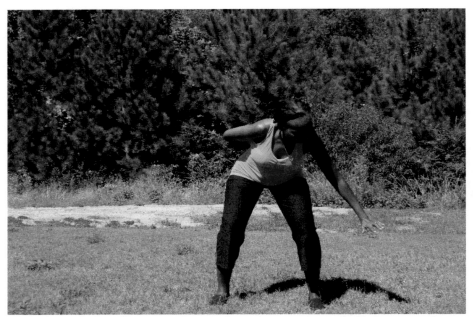

Exhale and visualize pressing an imaginary energy ball down to the ground with your left palm.

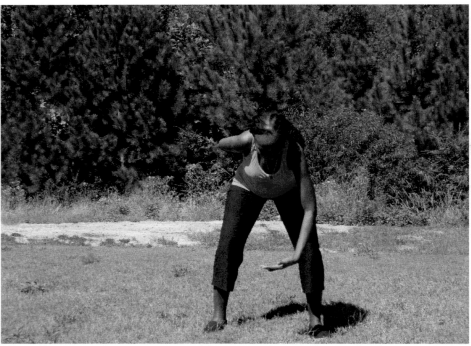

Visualize scooping up water with your palm while continuing to exhale.

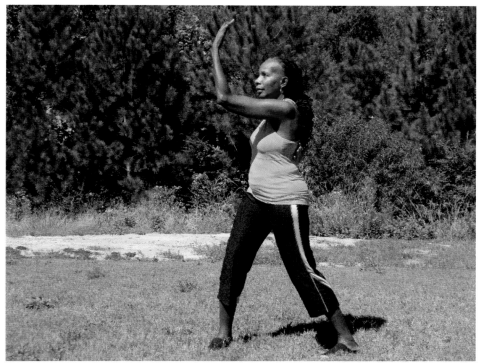
Visualize pouring water on your face to complete your exhalation

Kidney Posture Activation Instructions

1. Begin by standing in Wu Qi with normal breathing
2. Inhale a deep royal blue light into the kidney while and placing one arm above your head and the other behind your back.
3. Lower your arm and torso and turn slightly to your side while exhaling
4. Squat and scoop your palm downward exhaling
5. Inhale and raise your same palm to head level and repeat this sequence 10 times.

<u>**Association**</u>

Organ – Kidneys/Bladder
Elements – Water
Season - Winter
Color - Royal Blue
Emotion- Fear/courage

Benefits

Improves all kidney meridian related functions This postures targets the ears, chronic low back pain, reproductive system and bladder. This posture supports primal kidney functions, which include sexual functions, brain power and structural integrity. Practice the liver posture more often during the winter seasons to help maintain balance and prevent low back pain.

Heart/Small Intestine

Activation with red light, smile into the organ/ tongue touches the upper middle palate.

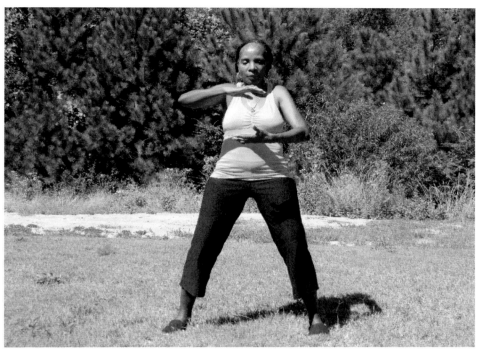

Form an imaginary energy/Qi ball with your hands.

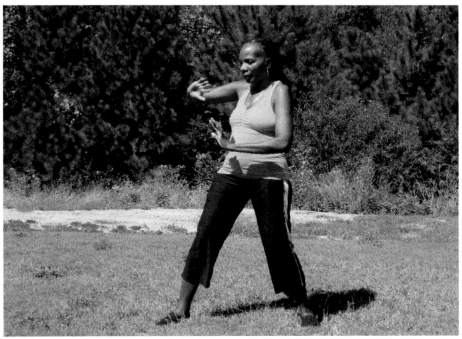

Begin to push the energy ball to your right side.

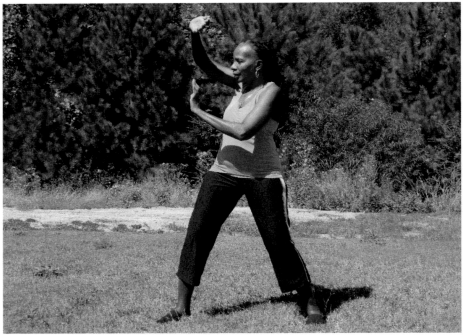
Lift the ball up to the level of your head.

The Heart Activation Instructions:
1. Start by standing while holding an imaginary energy ball and inhaling red light into the heart.
2. Move both hands to the side in a lifting and pushing type of movement. Exhale as you push out and inhale as you draw your hands inward.
3. Continue to raise both of your hands above to head level.
4. Return your hands to the energy ball holding position.
5. Perform the same sequence on the opposite side.
Repeat the entire sequence 10 times.

Association
Organ – Heart/Small Intestine
Elements – Fire
Season - Summer
Color – Red
Emotion – Joy/Hate

Benefits
Helps to improve the function of the heart, such as blood circulation, lowers blood pressure, headaches and compassion.   Practice the Heart posture more often during the summer and late summer seasons to keep your blood flowing smoothly, lower blood pressure and reduce stress.

Chapter 15

Opening the Spleen

Spleen/Stomach

Activate with /yellow light, smile into the organ/tongue touches the bottom gums behind the teeth.

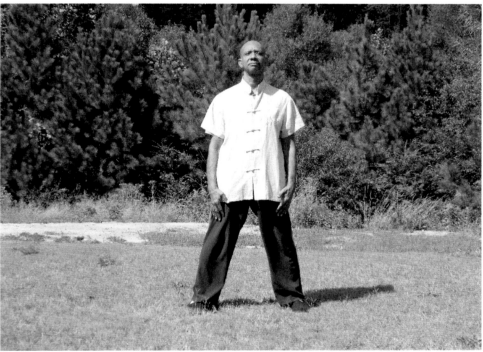

Stand in Wu Qi looking forward then lift your arms up from your center.

The spleen and stomach both represent the earth element and is responsible for building flesh and nourishing the body. Without a healthy spleen qi our bodies are unable to extract proper nutrients from our food, The stomach processes our food to a more soluble form for digestion This is a yang function. The spleen tends to store the energy processed which is more of a yin function.

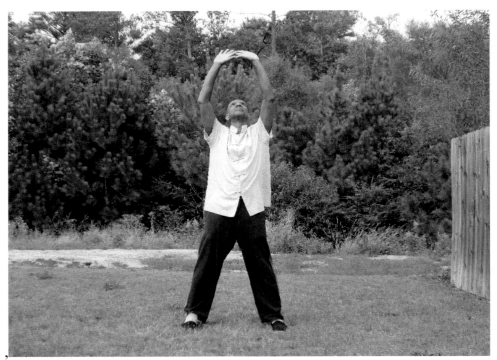

Inhale the sun's yellow bright light into the spleen and lift arms above head forming a triangle with your palms.

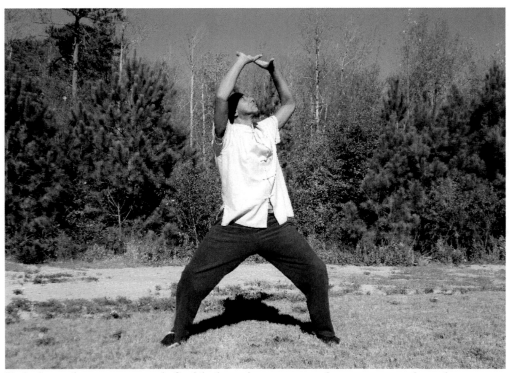

Exhale and turn to your left side keeping arms and at an upward angle. hips stationary and centered. Only the waist and arms should turn.

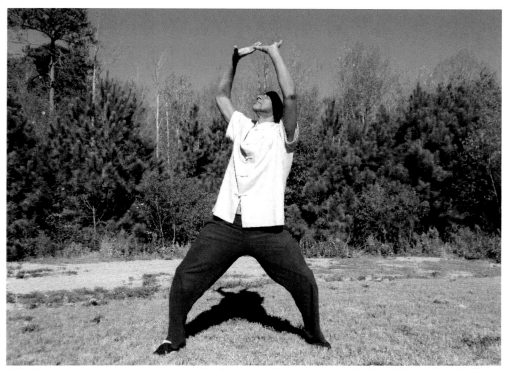

Inhale and return to the center before turning to your right side and exhaling. End the spleen sequence facing center.

Spleen Activation Instructions

See captions above for photos. Perform the complete sequence 5-10 times. Close out this sequence by inhaling, returning to center, exhaling and lowering your arms down the front torso back to the Wu Qi Standing Posture you began with.

Association

Organ – Spleen/Stomach
Element – Metal
Season – Late Summer
Color – Yellow
Emotion – Worry/Contentment

Benefits

This posture helps to improve digestion, blood sugar levels, stomach pH and balances the emotion of worrying or over thinking. Practice the spleen posture more often during the late summer seasons to help maintain balance and prevent stomach problems.

These 5 organ sequences complete the basic 5 Yin Organs Qigong set. When concluding your practice, we also recommend finishing up doing the Golden Turtle Back Qigong Posture for to its multiple benefits.

Due to the difficulty of this posture and the maximum pressure on the legs, we advise that you modify the posture to avoid any extreme discomforts until you are able enough to do it at the advance level. This sequence can be modified by not squatting too low if you have leg or hip problems.

The photos on the next page demonstrates how the posture at the advance level should be done.

Chapter 16

The Golden Turtle

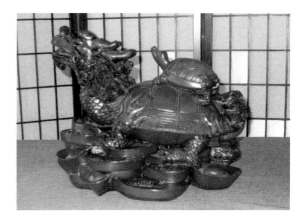

The Golden Turtle Immersing Itself in Water (Yang Position)

Golden Turtle Back Qigong Posture
Visualize a deep royal blue light, act and feel determined when doing this posture/tongue is on the upper palate.

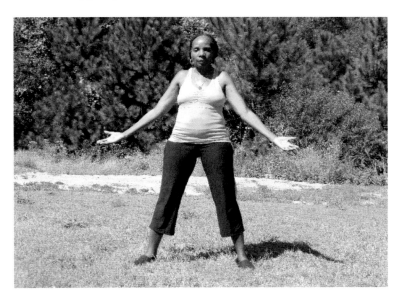

Raise your arms up from the sides while inhaling deep royal blue light into the kidneys with a strong determined focus.

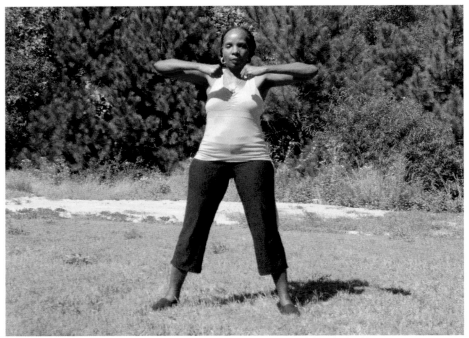

Tighten your forearms and lift your rib cage while inhaling.

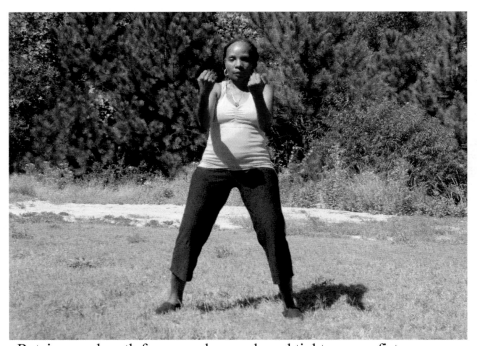

Retain your breath for several seconds and tighten your fists.

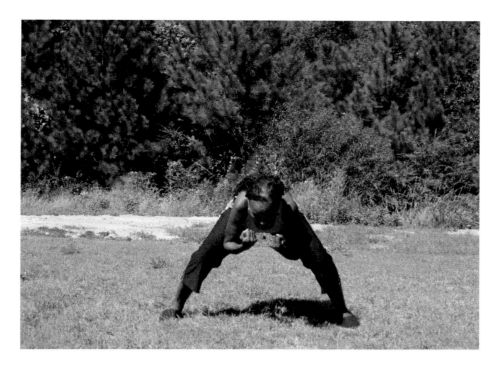

Lower yourself to a full squat position looking down exhaling 8 times in a rapid blacksmith bellow like breathing pattern while squeezing the anal sphincter muscle.

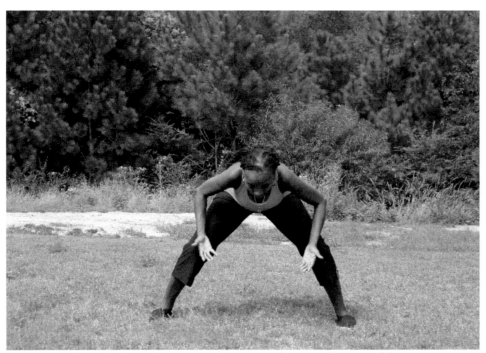

Relax and inhale deeply as you rise up to the standing position

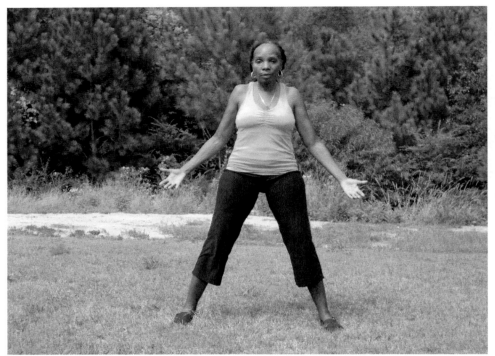

Pause and breathe normally for two cycles before starting again
The turtle sequence should be repeated for 3-5 sets.

Take precaution and follow direction carefully when practicing this posture gain a better over-standing on how to perform the Golden Turtle (Iron Shirt Qi Gong). If you are not strong enough limit your repetitions and avoid squatting too low. This is a more of an extreme position for many.

Side View

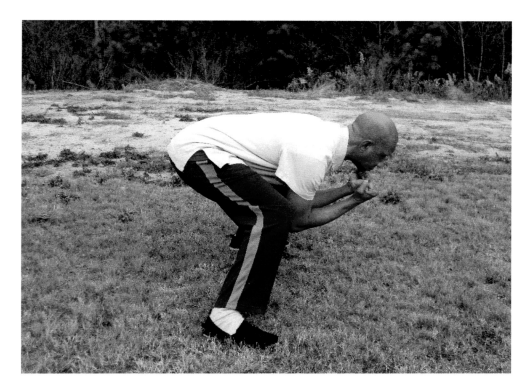

Dr. Isom side view of the Golden Turtle Posture done in the low position.

[Build Strength and Inner Fire]

Benefits

The Golden Turtle energizes the toes and all the tendons of the toes and the fasciae of the thighs and legs, and strengthens the back fasciae, spinal cord, sacrum, kidneys, adrenal glands, neck and head. This position anabolic in nature is also called the "Turtle Back". This posture can be practice more often during the winter and spring seasons because it is a yang posture that produces a lot of heat in the body.

Chapter 17

How to End your Qigong Session Properly

Once you have completed the final posture you should close out your Qigong session by sealing in all the energy that was circulated your body into the lower Dan Tien for storage. This area serves a reservoir storage tank for excess energy and can be withdrawn from when needed for healing or emergency fight or flight situations. The tongue is disconnected and suspended between the lower and upper palate.

How to Close and Seal in your Qi

To seal your energy back into your navel you will need to do a self- abdominal massage. Place your right palm on top of your left for men 3 fingers below your navel. Spiral out with your palms from the middle of your navel 9 times, until the top of the spiral ends at the base of your sternum at the 12 o'clock position. Then reverse, coming back in to the center of the navel in 6 spirals.

Place your palms over your navel, left first for men, right first for women, and concentrate your energy and attention there. Try to monitor how you are feeling.

Men and woman should do this in opposite directions as follows while keeping your tongue tip on the roof of your mouth.

Men spiral-out to the left/counterclockwise, and women spiral-out to the right/clockwise. When you have reached the limit of your sternum at 12 o'clock after 9 spirals, reverse direction to come back into the center of your navel in 6 spirals. Another optional ratio is 36 spirals in one directions followed by 24 spirals in reverse.

It is important to remember to disconnect your tongue. This disconnects the Governor and the Conception Channels. It is essential to do this when you are ending your practice to avoid feeling too energized to relax or sleep.

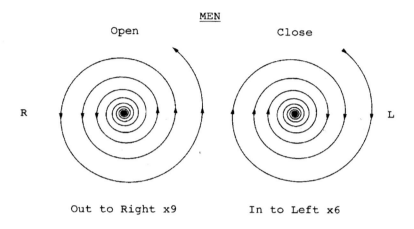

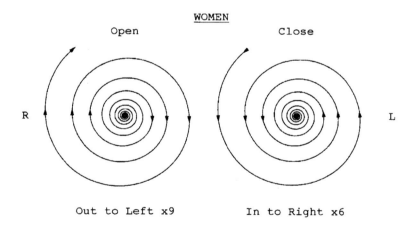

This concludes our **Life is Healing Qigong Level I 5 Yin Organs Qigong.** In the future, we hope to be able to offer training on Level II Which will focus on cleansing and purging the body of energetic and emotional toxins. Don't forget to visit our websites:

lifeishealing.com / harmonizingfist.com / **https://www.mydoterra.com/lifeishealing/#/**

**How to Become A
Qigong Therapist**

Successful completion and study of level I is required for those who are interested in a certification. Once completed a student will then become eligible to complete more advanced levels and standards for certification as a **Life is Healing Qigong Therapist**. Our certified qigong therapist will also become part of our historical lineage family tree and maintain high standards of practice as sanctioned by our school.

" Age is measured not in years but in lifetimes"

{NAMASTE}

(The spirit in me honors the spirit in you)

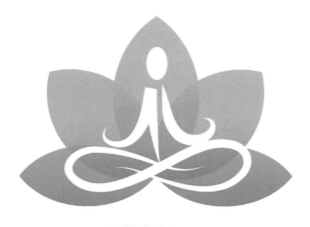

If you like to receive our free monthly newsletter send us an email at
lifeishealing@yahoo.com

For more information visit:
harmonizingfist.com
mydoterra.com/lifeishealing

Useful References

Chi Kung - Cultivating Personal Energy James MacRitchie. ISBN: 1862040648

The Roots of Chinese Qigong
Dr. Yang Jwing Ming ISBN: 1-886959-50-7

Chi Kung - Energy For Life
James MacRitchie. ISBN: 0007145683

Traditional Chinese Acupuncture: Meridians and Points
J.R. Worsley. ISBN: 090654003

The Complete Book of Chinese Health and Healing by Daniel Reid"
The Tao Of Health, Sex, and Longevity by Daniel Reid, Copy Right 1989,
ISBN 0-671-64811-X
Dr. Andrew Weils
http://www.drweil.com/health-wellness/balanced-living/wellness-therapies/qigong/

I Ching or Book of Changes. Richard Wilhelm. ISBN: 069109750

Tao Te Ching
Stephen Mitchell. ISBN: 0060812451

The Kings Medicine Cabinet by Dr. Josh Axe,
The Essential Life A Guide to Living
The Wellness Lifestyle 2nd Edition

(Excerpt from 'Inward Training' (Nei-Yeh), a poem found in the Kuan Tzu,
The Original Tao. translated by Harold D Roth, a text which the author
thinks may predate the Tao Te Ching.)

Made in the
USA
Lexington, KY